Items should be returned on or before the last date
shown below. Items not already requested by other
borrowers may be renewed in person, in writing or by
telephone. To renew, please quote the number on the
barcode label. To renew online a PIN is required.
This can be requested at your local library.
Renew online @ **www.dublincitypubliclibraries.ie**
Fines charged for overdue items will include postage
incurred in recovery. Damage to or loss of items will
be charged to the borrower. 610

Leabharlanna Poiblí Chathair Bhaile Átha Cliath
Dublin City Public Libraries

Date Due	Date Due	Date Due
	1 6 NOV 2018	

by the same authors

Personalisation and Dementia
A Guide for Person-Centred Practice
Helen Sanderson and Gill Bailey
Foreword by Jeremy Hughes
ISBN 978 1 84905 379 2
eISBN 978 0 85700 734 6

Making Individual Service Funds Work for
People with Dementia Living in Care Homes
How it Works in Practice
Helen Sanderson and Gill Bailey
With Lisa Martin
Foreword by Dr Sam Bennett
ISBN 978 1 84905 545 1
eISBN 978 0 85700 975 3

Person-Centred Teams
A Practical Guide to Delivering Personalisation
Through Effective Team-work
Helen Sanderson and Mary Beth Lepkowsky
ISBN 978 1 84905 455 3
eISBN 978 0 85700 830 5

The Individual Service Funds Handbook
Implementing Personal Budgets
in Provider Organisations
Helen Sanderson and Robin Miller
ISBN 978 1 84905 423 2
eISBN 978 0 85700 792 6

Creating Person-Centred Organisations
Strategies and Tools for Managing Change in
Health, Social Care and the Voluntary Sector
Stephen Stirk and Helen Sanderson
ISBN 978 1 84905 260 3
eISBN 978 0 85700 549 6

A Practical Guide to Delivering
Personalisation
Person-Centred Practice in Health and Social Care
Helen Sanderson and Jaimee Lewis
ISBN 978 1 84905 194 1
eISBN 978 0 85700 422 2

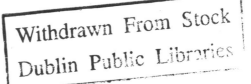
Person-Centred Thinking with Older People

6 Essential Practices

HELEN SANDERSON, HELEN BOWN AND GILL BAILEY

FOREWORDS BY DOROTHY RUNNICLES AND DAVID BRINDLE

Jessica Kingsley *Publishers*
London and Philadelphia

Photographs by Eddie Philips.
Graphics by Julie Barclay.

First published in 2015
by Jessica Kingsley Publishers
73 Collier Street
London N1 9BE, UK
and
400 Market Street, Suite 400
Philadelphia, PA 19106, USA

www.jkp.com

Library of Congress Cataloging in Publication Data
Sanderson, Helen, 1965- , author.
  Person-centred thinking with older people : six essential practices
/ Helen Sanderson, Helen Bown, and Gill Bailey ; foreword by
David Brindle and Dorothy Runnicles. -- Second edition.
      p. ; cm.
  Includes bibliographical references and index.
  ISBN 978-1-84905-612-0 (alk. paper)
  I. Bown, Helen, 1967- , author. II. Bailey, Gill, author. III. Title.
  [DNLM: 1. Patient-Centered Care--methods. 2. Aged.
3. Personality. 4. Professional-Patient Relations.
WT 31]
  R733
  610--dc23
                          2014041983

British Library Cataloguing in Publication Data
A CIP catalogue record for this book is available from the British Library

ISBN 9781849056120
eISBN 9781784500825

Printed and bound in China

CONTENTS

Foreword

As an older person approaching my 90th birthday and a service user of domiciliary social care for more than a decade, I am privileged to be asked to give my views about this book. Sadly, from my experience I have not had the opportunity to test out the approach so well described within it. It has not been used by any of the agencies that have provided services to me. But, as the eligibility criteria preclude me from grant aid – like 80 per cent of older people – I have established ways of achieving some degree of personal control over the support I get from a circle of friends, neighbours, family members and professional workers.

However, at the moment I can still see, hear and write, so communication is reasonably easy for me. I have many friends with disabilities that make them less able to exercise choice, voice or control. For these people, their opportunities to improve their lives require a willingness and enthusiasm on the part of the service provider and this book illustrates possibilities.

This book describes an approach and not a service. An essential element of this approach is about ways of communicating.

Major communication problems occur for some users of services: for example, workers who have little knowledge or understanding of the English language. For some people, good communication can be achieved by body language, emotional and empathy links.

But for others, better communication with users is not on the agenda. Many of us can give examples from our experiences, where in reality few choices were available – even with the food supply, despite a wide written menu. Theoretically, these choices existed, but they were not implemented. Systems can be perverted when the monitoring of outcomes with the customers is not in place.

The use of these tools could be an exciting development that could change people's lives. The challenge then is to turn these useful tools into wider action.

Dorothy Runnicles

Foreword

None of us is getting any younger, but more of us are getting much older than ever in the history of humankind. The ageing of society is an astonishing gift, presenting us in the UK with an average 30 more years of life than was enjoyed by our great grandparents. One in three, perhaps one in two, babies born today can expect to live beyond 100.

But older age brings challenge as well as opportunity. To lead rich and rewarding lifestyles in our later years, many of us will need care and support. And having grown up in an increasingly consumerist era, we shall want and expect choice and control over that help: who provides it, when it is provided and, most critically, how it is provided. The days of take-it-or-leave-it services are over.

This book shows how to give older people true choice and control by not just asking them what they want, ticking a box marked consultation, but by involving them fully in planning their care and support as an integral part of their preferred routine. Not so much a service, more a way of life.

People's stories told in these pages demonstrate vividly what is possible when person-centred thinking is fully applied. And these are stories not only of people living independently, but also of people living in residential settings and living with disabilities and dementia. The onset of a debilitating condition does not bring with it any automatic forfeit of rights to voice, choice or control.

Much has changed since the first edition of this book appeared, not least the global recession and the unprecedented austerity regime in the UK that has hollowed out so many of our public services. Are person-centred thinking and practices unaffordable luxuries in the harsh new world? By no means. If anything, the realities of a fresh settlement between the citizen and the state, and between the citizen and their community, call for even greater emphasis on moulding care and support around the needs of the individual – and their assets. Everyone has something to contribute.

Recent exposures of poor and harmful practice in traditional care services have prompted a focus on lack of compassion on the part of care-givers. That is an important response, but being kinder and more respectful of dignity is only half the answer to the underlying problem. The other half is to embed a far greater understanding of, and respect for, the rights of the older person, their character and their preferences.

Each of us is unique. It is incumbent upon care professionals, family carers and friends and neighbours to know us, and what is important to us, as we age. Person-centred thinking can cultivate that knowledge.

David Brindle
Public services editor, *The Guardian*

ACKNOWLEDGEMENTS

Thank you to the people who helped make this book possible.

Thank you to Arthur Jones, Hilda Williams, Beatrice Cooper, Julie Moore, Margaret Holden and Carolyn Aston for generously sharing your experience and stories, and to the staff at Tameside Council. We also appreciate the help given by Steve Mycroft, Sheila Mannion, Dawn Frost, Carol Saint, Cathy Smith and everyone who lives and works at Oakwood House, Stalybridge, Tameside.

Thank you to Cath Barton, Lynda and Alan for sharing their Community Circle story.

The Older People's Programme is now the Ageing and Older People's Programme at the National Development Team for Inclusion. NDTi would like to thank all those people who have shared their stories and insights through the Circles of Support project working with people living with dementia in Devon, Dorset, Hampshire and West London. Particular thanks go to Alison Macadam who led the Circles project and wrote up the stories; the local partners involved in each area; and Nada and Rachael from Innovations in Dementia.

The story of Mary's person-centred review is extracted from *Personalisation and Dementia* by Helen Sanderson and Gill Bailey, 2013, published by Jessica Kingsley Publishers.

The materials on person-centred thinking were developed by The Learning Community for Person Centred Practices and are used with permission.

To learn more about person-centred practices please go to:

www.learningcommunity.us

www.helensandersonassociates.co.uk

Photographs by Eddie Philips, graphics by Julie Barclay.

Introduction

This book is about using person-centred thinking to enable older people to have much greater control and say over what they need and want in order to be full and active citizens, whatever their support needs, wherever they live, whoever they live with and however they live.

It is an updated version of the *Practicalities and Possibilities* book that we wrote together in 2007.[1] This edition provides additional information and material developed since that time, including new stories and examples of person-centred practices with older people from the last seven years.

This new edition also takes account of and reflects the changing times, including the impact of the 2008 global economic crash and subsequent era of austerity on both the public and commercial sectors in the UK and beyond, including services and supports for older people. The formation of a Conservative and Liberal Democrat coalition government in 2010 led to changes to services and supports in the UK, with new policies, legislative and regulatory frameworks. We also saw the tragic consequences of abuse and poor practice within services and care settings where older and disabled people live, for example at Mid Staffordshire General Hospital and at Winterbourne View. These examples highlight more than ever the imperative of ensuring that person-centred practices and support become the everyday norm rather than an isolated innovation.

---

1   Bowers, H., Bailey, G., Sanderson, H., Easterbrook, L. and Macadam, A. (2007) *Person Centred Thinking with Older People: Practicalities and Possibilities.* Stockport, UK: HSA Press.

This introductory chapter outlines some of these changes and contemporary issues, identifying where person-centred thinking tools and practices can make a positive difference to older people's lives through the support they experience. It summarises both what these changes are, and work that has taken place to keep person-centred practices at the forefront of service improvements for older people.

In the first edition, we talked about the work that had been done – especially over the preceding ten years – to develop person-centred approaches in health and social care services in order to deliver better treatment and care for older people. We reflected that, in spite of these developments, very often services were actually doing things in a more efficient and organised way rather than really doing them differently, in ways that make sense for older people.

We also recognised that older people have commitments, roles and responsibilities that define them and shape their need for support in much broader ways than are taken account of by traditional services. Person-centred thinking and practices ensure that older people are supported in ways that make sense to them, and at the same time can deliver better, more efficient services that improve their lives and life chances.

There are opportunities, therefore, for showing how person-centred practices improve things for older people, and for services and agencies too. Person-centred practices are not a luxury add-on; they need to be central to all care and support across the spectrum of public and privately funded services that many older people rely on every day.

Whilst this automatically means that we are talking about a much broader, and more exciting, range of developments and ways of working, it can also seem daunting for professionals who are involved in providing and commissioning services. That is one of the reasons that we wanted to write this book and feel it is still relevant today.

Why this book matters to us

Our work at the Older People's Programme (now the Ageing and Older People's Programme at the National Development Team for Inclusion, NDTi) and Helen Sanderson Associates brings us into contact with a diverse range of older people, family and other social networks (neighbours, colleagues, friends, wider communities, volunteers), professionals, services and agencies.

We originally decided to develop our ideas and experiences into a practical book because of four issues that we were familiar with from our work. These four issues still resonate today, and person-centred thinking and practices can help to address them.

1. First, we observed what happens to people's lives if services come to be the dominant part – whether in terms of where someone lives, the arrangement of their daily lives or the people with whom they have contact. We still often meet older people who are living in two worlds – a 'service world' and 'ordinary life'. Most of their contact is with people who are either paid for providing a particular role or who have a formal volunteering relationship. It is often their 'ordinary life' and their ordinary social networks that shrink – and their 'care life' or 'support life' with its 'formal' network that now dominates. Particular problems can arise for older people and their families when the service world starts to dominate and not support or make room for their 'ordinary life'. This shrinking is most likely to happen when someone's situation suddenly and dramatically changes. It can also happen gradually and almost imperceptibly over time. In older age, the most common reasons for sudden change like this tend to be illness, disability, bereavement, divorce or moving to a new place. But the way people have lived their lives in younger years may also be having an impact now. For example, someone may have lived happily with a very small circle or social network of close friends

and relatives, but if some of these people have now died or are themselves ill there may be fewer and fewer people to call on or do things with.

2. We are also often struck by how many older people tell us that they have been told to (for example) 'come to day care because I was lonely' – but who, when asked, say they are still lonely even though they now regularly attend a day centre or lunch club. Some services, at least, seem to us to be more about a transaction than about transforming someone's life. In other words, there is greater emphasis on delivering something than on making sure that what is delivered is addressing the need or the gap(s) identified by the person. There has been an increasing recognition of the impact of loneliness and isolation for people of all ages, and particularly for some older people whose networks and relationships shrink or change (e.g. through the Campaign to End Loneliness). We believe that thinking about people as individuals, taking account of their histories, past as well as present (and possible future) relationships, gifts and talents as well as their needs, can help to deliver support that enables and empowers them to make positive changes in their lives. Just providing services for one part of a day or aspect of someone's life will not make them less lonely or less isolated. Changing the way we think about that person and what they are capable of achieving, contributing and doing could help them feel valued, appreciated and connected to the wider world around them. We also think that circles of support (e.g. Community Circles) have a contribution here.

3. The third set of issues was highlighted by older people taking part in a stakeholder conference called Living Well in Later Life[2]. This event brought together people from

---

2   Bowers, H., Mendonca, P. and Easterbrook, L. (2002) 'Living well in later life – an agenda for national and local action', Conference Report. York, UK: Joseph Rowntree Foundation.

diverse backgrounds to think about what a good later life looks like. Participants identified seven dimensions to living well in later life:

a) being active, staying healthy and contributing

b) continuing to learn

c) friends and community – being valued and belonging

d) the importance of family and relationships

e) valuing diversity

f) approachable local services

g) having choices, taking risks.

4. The order shown reflects the priorities shared by those who participated in the event. Whilst this will clearly differ for everyone – all of us have very different ideas about what's important to us – it is interesting to note that all participants placed services and issues of risk last!

5. Key among the seven elements is the importance of relationships and networks. This isn't just about having a list of people you see or speak with – it is crucially about the quality and nature of those relationships and contacts, including how time is spent with them.

6. This issue in particular has struck us time and again, and we can't state strongly enough how vital it is to have people in your life with whom you have good, close relationships and with whom you do certain things that are important to you and to them.

7. Person-centred care has been a key focus of developments in health and social care for older people since the introduction of the Department of Health's National Service Framework for Older People in 2001, which

highlights it in Standard Two. Subsequent publications and guidance over the 13 years since have continued to emphasise the importance of being person-centred, and of developing person-centred services and responses to older people's needs. The policy and practice round-up on pages 18–20 summarises the raft of recent policy and practice frameworks, each referencing person-centred approaches, personalisation and social capital – in other words, the assets, strengths and networks that people bring to their own and others' support and services. It follows, therefore, that older people's networks and relationships are integral to successful implementation of these frameworks. As one participant at the Living Well in Later Life conference put it: 'We are part of the solution, not the problem'.

8. This brings us onto the fourth key issue. Many professionals and staff working in different agencies across the public, private and voluntary sectors tell us they are 'already doing person-centred care'. By this they often seem to mean that they are asking older people what they want, or anticipating what they might want, but often without really involving and engaging them as equal partners and valued citizens. Many more people are engaged in discussions and decisions about their own care and support as well as wider service developments (increasingly through processes and techniques collectively known as 'co-production'). However, there are equally many older people who need support in their lives whose voices are not well heard or influential.

9. Working Together for Change is one example of an approach that engages individuals, families, staff and decision makers in reviewing what's working and not working in local support, and identifying the changes that need to happen in the future.[3]

---

3   See www.helensandersonassociates.co.uk for more information.

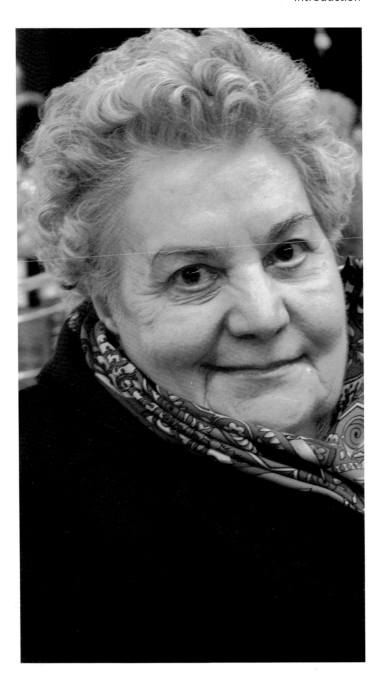

Contemporary issues in social policy and practice

Working with older people in enabling and person-centred ways has always been important, but particular aspects of the current policy and practice environments make it a high priority, and more people, agencies and influential bodies are ready to listen and learn than ever before. We highlight three big reasons for driving forward with person-centred approaches with older people now.

One of the main reasons is that as we design and develop a health and social care system fit for the future, we must recognise that the largest group of people affected by this system will be older people. This is especially true when it comes to developments relating to self-directed support, or personalisation. Person-centred thinking skills and practices offer a different approach to thinking not only about services, but also about older people and ageing more widely.

Second, the policy landscape looks quite different today from the one we described in the first edition seven years ago. Much has happened to enshrine and promote personalisation and different approaches to delivering services in person-centred ways. At the same time, the wider agenda around ageing and older people has become narrower and less well defined. There is no current strategy on ageing and the focus within policy is largely on reforming care and support and pensions. Whilst these are important, not least because of problems experienced within services and reduced public service budgets (and therefore service provision), this means that the wider issues and priorities of our ageing population are not clearly on decision makers' radars. We reflected in the first edition on the need to understand the varied characteristics of our ageing population, and why and how individuals age differently, especially with respect to their health, wellbeing and disability – and on their need for different kinds of support. We believe this is as true today as it was in 2007.

Third, we wrote seven years ago about older people's aspirations, and their rights and demands for equality, choice and greater control regardless of their need for support on a day-to-day basis. The Equality Act 2010 introduced a new legal duty on all public bodies to ensure and demonstrate that their services are 'age equal'; in other words, that their services do not discriminate on the basis of age. It brought together all previous equalities legislation under one umbrella and this new requirement on age was a landmark, ensuring that age discrimination is now illegal.[4]

What do older people typically experience from services?

- Fragmented services and support between different agencies, departments, services and teams.

- The health and social care world dominates, and crisis care dominates above all – other parts of life can often appear to fade away, even though they are central to wellbeing, self-esteem and health (e.g. family life and other relationships, being active and contributing, having a role and purpose, etc.).

- Choice is restricted and support is still largely traditional in nature, especially for older people with high support needs.

- Access to and experience of personal budgets is increasing, but is still low overall and in some places is extremely underdeveloped. There are important lessons about what helps, what gets in the way and what matters to older people in taking control of the resources that relate to

---

4   An online resource, 'Achieving Age Equality in Health and Social Care' provides evidence-based criteria and practical ways of looking at services in partnership with older people, to end age discrimination and make progress towards age equality. This includes references to working in person-centred ways and adopting person-centred approaches for making this happen (see http://age-equality.southwest.nhs.uk for more information).

their support (as set out in the guide *Putting People First: Personal budgets and older people – making it happen*[5]), yet all too often these lessons have not been widely implemented.

- Whilst there are many positive stories about older people shaping and controlling their own support shared in this book, we know that some older people are very marginalised and excluded from decisions about their support. For example, older people with mental health difficulties, people living with dementia, older people who live in care homes, older people from black and minority ethnic communities, lesbian, gay and transgender older people, and those with complex needs.

We're reminded of these typical experiences again through the Practicalities and Possibilities Development Programme. It highlights seven lessons for embedding person-centred approaches:

1. Involve older people from the start – both in their own support and in wider service developments and strategic decisions. Reach out and engage those whose voices are not well heard to ensure they can also fully participate.

2. Partnerships underpin success: think creatively about your partners and ensure they reflect the whole of older people's lives rather than their experiences of services alone.

3. Join it all up and commit to making this happen at a senior, strategic level. Change will not happen and be sustained on the ground and in people's lives if decision makers and commissioners don't sign up to making it happen at the top.

4. Well-connected leaders with clear values make change happen – inspire and support your teams and colleagues to

---

5   Department of Health (2009) *Putting People First: Personal budgets and older people – making it happen.* London, UK: Department of Health. Available online at: www.ndti.org.uk/uploads/files/PSSOP.pdf.

adopt person-centred approaches and watch them flourish and grow.

5. Invest in creating the right conditions for change rather than assuming person-centred practices will happen on their own because they're 'a good thing'. Some people will need persuading and others will need convincing and everyone will need to know that working in this way makes a difference to older people and local services.

6. Recognise this is a change for everyone (older people and families as well as staff) and support people at every stage, ensuring people are equipped and enabled to work in new ways and change practices and systems if they need to.

7. Take a problem-solving approach that celebrates success, recognises and values contributions and focuses on 'what we can do' rather than what's getting in the way.

What are the main developments in policy and practice?

Box I.1 summarises some of the most important current policy and practice frameworks, highlighting key changes since 2007, and the increased and ongoing focus on personalised support and service responses.

Box I.1 Person-centred policy and practice summary

Here are the most important current policy and practice frameworks. The list highlights key changes since 2007 and the increased and ongoing focus on personalisation.

Putting People First (2008)[6] – The first health and social care policy framework setting out key requirements and deliverables on personalised care and support for all adults.

Delivering Lifetime Homes, Lifetime Neighbourhoods (2008)[7] – A vision for affordable, accessible housing and options for housing-related support with a key focus on choice, based on older people's priorities and preferences.

Independent Living Strategy, 2008 (superseded by Fulfilling Potential, 2013)[8] – The government's commitment to increasing the voice, choice and control of disabled people of all ages by 2025.

Making a Strategic Shift towards Prevention and Early Intervention (2008)[9] – Part of the suite of publications

---

6   Department of Health (2008), *Putting People First: A shared vision and commitment to the transformation of Adult Social Care.* London, UK: Department of Health. Available online at: http://webarchive.nationalarchives.gov. uk/20130107105354/http://www.dh.gov.uk/prod_consum_dh/groups/ dh_digitalassets/@dh/@en/documents/digitalasset/dh_081119.pdf.

7   Department for Communities and Local Government (2008) *Delivering Lifetime Homes, Lifetime Neighbourhoods.* London, UK: Department for Communities and Local Government. Available at http://webarchive.nationalarchives. gov.uk/20120919132719/http:/www.communities.gov.uk/documents/ housing/pdf/deliveringlifetimehomes.pdf.

8   Office for Disability Issues (2013) *Fulfilling Potential: Improving the Lives of Disabled People.* London, UK: Office for Disability Issues. Available at www. gov.uk/government/collections/fulfilling-potential-working-together-to- improve-the-lives-of-disabled-people.

9   Department of Health (2008) *Making a Strategic Shift Towards Prevention and Early Intervention.* London, UK: Department of Health. Available at http:// webarchive.nationalarchives.gov.uk/20081202170926/networks.csip.org. uk/prevention.

connected to Putting People First, demonstrating how health and social care services can enable resources to be diverted from secondary acute care and long-term care to earlier intervention and a broader range of creative supports.

Personal Budgets and Older People – Making it Happen (2009)[10] – Practical guidance setting out the building blocks for delivering personalised care and support with and for older people, including a key chapter on person-centred approaches and coproduction (see below).

Personalisation: Don't Just Do It, Coproduce and Live It. A Guide to Coproduction with Older People (2009)[11] – A practical guide to coproduction with older people including definitions on what it is and practical examples and steps for achieving real voice and influence in decision making.

The formation of the Think Local Act Personal (TLAP) partnership in 2011,[12] bringing together more than 30 organisations committed to transforming health and care through personalisation and community-based support; *and the development of the Making it Real statements*, setting out what people who use services and carers expect if support services are truly personalised.

National Dementia Strategy, 2009–2014,[13] including a renewed, refreshed strategy from 2014 onwards, aimed at improving diagnosis, care and support for people living with dementia whilst tackling the stigma and discrimination often faced.

---

10 Department of Health (2009) *Personal Budgets and Older People – Making it Happen*. London, UK: Department of Health. Available at www.ndti.org.uk/uploads/files/PSSOP.pdf.

11 Archibald, A., Barker, S. and Barry, J. (2009) *Personalisation – don't just do it – co-produce it and live it! A guide to co-production with older people.* Christchurch, Dorset and Stockport: National Development Team for Inclusion and Helen Sanderson Associates (HSA).

12 See www.thinklocalactpersonal.org.uk for further information.

13 Department of Health (2009-2014) *Living Well with Dementia: A National Dementia Strategy.* London, UK: Department of Health. Available at www.gov.uk/government/publications/living-well-with-dementia-a-national-dementia-strategy.

> *The Better Life Programme at Joseph Rowntree Foundation*[14] *ran from 2009–2013* – It explored ways of increasing the voice, choice and control of older people with high support needs, as a result of research findings on older people's vision for long term care (OPP 2009) that highlighted the pressing need to transform people's experiences if they have or develop high support needs.
>
> *The Equality Act 2010 and supporting Equality Strategy (2011)*[15] legally protect people from discrimination in the workplace and wider society, replacing previous anti-discriminatory laws with a single Act. It bans age discrimination against adults in the provision of services and public functions.
>
> *Caring for Our Future: Reforming Care and Support White Paper (2012)*[16]*; precursor to the Care Act 2014, Department of Health* – Sets out reformed care and support arrangements spanning assessments through to the funding and provision of long-term care. The primary focus is on personalised assessments and care and support planning, choice and control through a diverse range of support options and greater emphasis on quality and outcomes in response to the Francis Inquiry Report.

This summary highlights that personalisation and adopting person-centred approaches at all levels of service delivery and development have been enshrined in government policy and in best practice guidance over the last decade, and indeed longer. Changes in government and the harsh financial climate have not pushed this commitment out of sight. The challenge

---

14   See www.jrf.org.uk/topic/betterlife?gclid=CLPG7e2smMICFWPmwgodPE sAbw.

15   See https://www.gov.uk/government/uploads/system/uploads/attachment_ data/file/85049/specific-duties.pdf for information on the Equality Act and Equality Strategy.

16   Department of Health (2012). *Caring for our Future: Reforming Care and Support.* Available online at https://www.gov.uk/government/uploads/system/ uploads/attachment_data/file/136422/White-Paper-Caring-for-our-future-reforming-care-and-support-PDF-1580K.pdf.

now is to enable and ensure that this happens for all older people when resources are scarce, development capacity to support change is limited, and wider welfare reforms raise other problems and challenges in people's lives.

Person-centred thinking tools

The stories and examples in this book come from our work in introducing and embedding person-centred practices with providers and councils, and from exploring circles of support, initially through the Circles project and now through Community Circles.[17]

Each of the following six chapters introduces and explains one core person-centred thinking tool and its practice, and shares older people's stories and examples of how it is used. At the end of each chapter we suggest where these tools could be used. These are the six tools in brief:

ONE-PAGE PROFILES

One-page profiles bring together appreciations of a person and reflect what is important to and for them. 'Important to' describes what really matters to the person, from their perspective. 'Important for' is about the help or support that they need to stay healthy, safe and well. Personalisation starts with the person, knowing who they are, what matters to them and how they want to be supported. A one-page profile therefore is the foundation of personalisation.

RELATIONSHIP CIRCLE

A relationship map or circle is a good way of identifying and capturing who is important to an older person, to ensure that there is at least one person and to actively seek to widen the connections and relationships that someone has.

---

17 See www.community-circles.co.uk and www.communitycirclesblog.wordpress.com.

COMMUNICATION CHARTS

The communication chart is a powerful and simple way to record how an older person communicates. This is critical if someone doesn't talk, and is also important where people only use a few words, or communicate most powerfully with their behaviours. It can also help if the person has memory or orientation problems, as in the case of people with dementias.

HISTORIES

Older people's histories can easily become lost or be left untold. A conscious effort to listen to and record individual histories can help staff to understand and appreciate people in a different way and, in doing so, develop different relationships with them.

WISHING

Older people may be keen to share and explore their own personal goals and dreams – their wishes.

WORKING AND NOT WORKING

Simply asking an older person what is working and not working in their life tells us so much. This information may be used to change what can be changed and to help us understand what really matters to people.

We end the book by exploring how these person-centred thinking tools provide the foundation for care and support planning, and within circles of support, and look forward to what may come next – both in terms of ongoing practice and service developments, and the broader contexts within which this work takes place.

We hope you find this book a useful resource in your work and your own lives – as individuals, family members, friends and neighbours who want the communities and places we live in to be good places to grow old.

Chapter 1
One-Page Profiles

The foundation of delivering person-centred support is a one-page profile. A one-page profile brings together what people appreciate about the person, and reflects what is important to and for them. It is vital that anyone supporting an older person knows what matters to them as an individual, and exactly how they want to be supported. In this chapter we introduce appreciations, and then look at a fundamental person-centred thinking skill – looking at what is important to and for someone, and how this is recorded in a one-page profile. We also describe two ways of getting started with a one-page profile – finding out about good days and bad days, and an informal one-page profile meeting.

Appreciations

Although in many cultures older people are honoured and revered for their wisdom and experience, in western society this is often not the case. The poem, 'Crabbit Old Woman'[1] by Phyllis McCormack (1996) reflects the way older people may be seen in hospital, and certainly how older people themselves feel they are seen.

A key aspect of person-centred practice is appreciation, and having a focus on what we like and admire about people. For many this is counter-cultural, and therefore we need to remind

---

1   The poem 'Crabbit Old Woman' was published by Phyllis McCormack. It was also found among the possessions of an aged lady who died on the geriatric ward of a hospital. It is also called 'What Do You See'.

ourselves how important appreciation is, and the difference it can make.

What we appreciate about someone is crucial for developing and building a relationship with them, so for staff, appreciation is a critical but often overlooked first step in getting to know someone and playing a part in the most intimate aspects of their life.

Appreciation can also help families and friends to rediscover their relationships with an older relative or neighbour, so it is important for maintaining and renewing the ties we all have with different people in our lives. This can be particularly helpful if someone has developed a dementia and has lost aspects of their memory or association with other people in their lives.

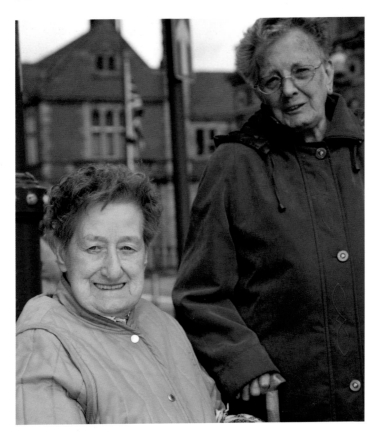

Asking ourselves what we appreciate about somebody can be a really good way of starting to work in a person-centred way. It helps us to take a step back and see who that person is, to appreciate their qualities and strengths, and to counter our tendency to focus on how much support an older person needs.

Mary Groves

Mary says she has had a great life. She is 91 and has lived at Oakwood House, a residential home with 17 other people, for the past two years. She says:

> I have a lot of living to do yet. I'm going anywhere until I'm at least 200!

She is happy and content, and likely to burst into song when you least expect it. Every Saturday, her sister and niece, Susan and Agnes, visit. Mary loves these visits. Staff asked Susan and Agnes to consider what they appreciate about Mary. Not many people are asked these questions about their relatives, and they were surprised and delighted to contribute.

This is what they came up with:

What we appreciate about Mary

- a fantastic, cheeky sense of humour

- an eternal optimist

- affectionate and loyal

- very nurturing

- sociable and caring

- infectious giggle

- very kind

- honest

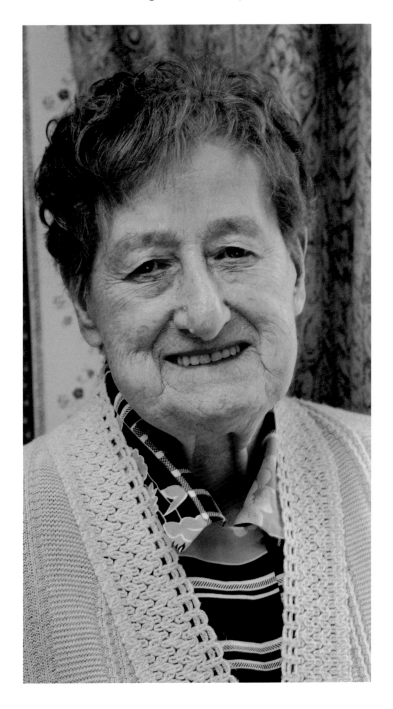

- laughs so easily

- the warmest person I know; you instantly care about her

- positive attitude and so funny

- always lifts my spirits

- feel better for talking with her

- a smashing character.

Mary glows as this list is read to her. She uses it to introduce herself to new members of staff, and says that it makes her 'feel loved and valued'.

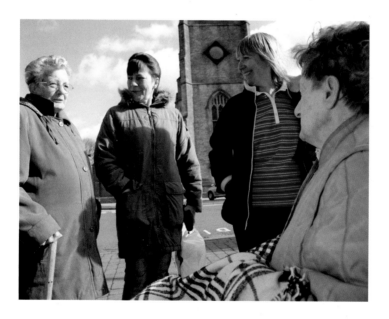

Important to and for

The fundamental person-centred thinking skill is being able to separate what is important *to* someone from what is important *for* them, and to find the balance between the two.

'Important to' is what really matters to the person, from their perspective. 'Important for' is about the help or support that they need to stay healthy, safe and well.

Services are usually very good at describing and delivering what is important for someone – for example what medication the person needs, how they must be positioned, how to make sure they are clean. If the older person needs a lot of support, especially on a daily basis, their nurse or carer may record this. Alternatively, the information may just be passed from carer to carer. What is usually missing in exchanges like this is what matters to the person, how they want their support provided and the balance between the two.

The managers of Oakwood House wanted to continue to improve the service that they offer people. They thought that one thing that they could change that would improve the quality of everyone's life would be to look at the evening routine at the home. They worked with all the staff to give them an understanding of and confidence in person-centred thinking skills. The staff worked with a person-centred planning co-ordinator and developed, with each individual in the home, a description of what was important to each person about their night-time routine, and what support each person needed (what was important for them). The managers then worked at making sure that what was important to each individual was happening so that people were getting support in the way that they wanted it.

Nora lives in Oakwood House and her story illustrates how to think about and discover what is important to someone and what is important for them.

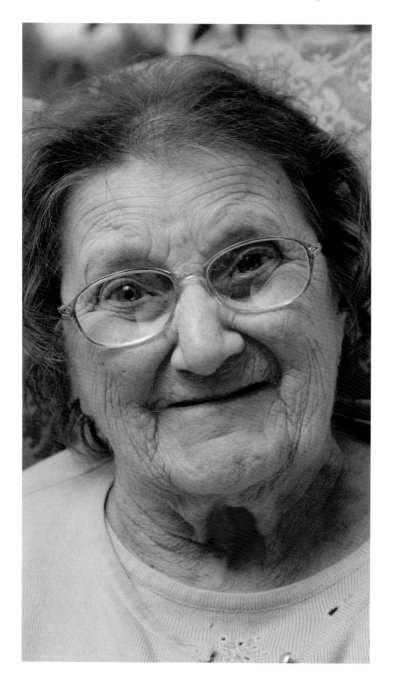

Nora Hughes

Nora is 87 years of age, and is a real character, full of chuckles and fun. She has a beautiful dress sense. She loves to see her children, Tony, Jim, Margaret and Irene.

What is important to Nora

Nora needs her routines to run like clockwork: everything has to happen at a certain time, otherwise this will develop into a bad evening and night for Nora.

It is really important to Nora that other people living at Oakwood House do not go into her bedroom, although she is happy for staff to do so. Nora must begin getting ready for bed at 7.30pm. As soon as the music comes on at the end of *Emmerdale*, Nora's favourite soap opera, she will take her feet off her footstool, remove the rug from her knee and look in an obvious way at the clock.

Nora washes her face herself using Dove soap. She loves to wear clean clothes each night for bed and must choose which nightie to wear. Nora also chooses the clothes she will wear the following day whilst getting ready for bed. Nora must have a body wash each evening in order to feel comfortable and clean for bed. She has talc on after her wash – no particular favourite, but usually scented. Nora loves her four pillows to be arranged comfortably once she is in bed. She is only comfy with lightweight covers and must have cotton sheets and a bedspread – she must not have a duvet! Nora loves her small lamp by the bed to stay on all night and the bedroom door to remain open.

What is important for Nora

Staff should acknowledge Nora's wish that other people living at Oakwood House do not go into her bedroom, and support her with this respectfully, by speaking to the other people living there when necessary.

Nora's reliance on routine is central to her happiness and staff need to be aware of her cues when she is ready to go to bed and respond – this will invariably be at 7.30pm. Two staff should support Nora from her armchair into her wheelchair to go to get ready for bed in her room. Nora needs support to use the commode in her room and she will then have a wash. Nora needs support in filling the sink with warm water and her flannel then needs to be soaped up with her Dove soap so that she can wash her face. The cloth then needs to be rinsed and handed back to Nora so she can rinse her face and she will then dry her face herself. Nora chooses from three nightdresses, which staff hold up – Nora will fix her eyes and say yes to the one she wishes to wear for bed. Nora always has clean underwear and pad for bed. Two staff should support Nora into bed and then arrange her four pillows comfortably around her. Nora's bedroom should always be warm enough for her to sleep comfortably with just a cotton sheet and bedspread. If it is very cold Nora may like a blanket. Nora's small lamp must be left on and her door open.

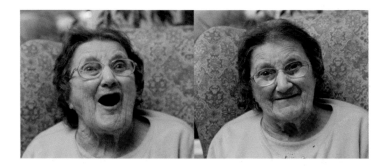

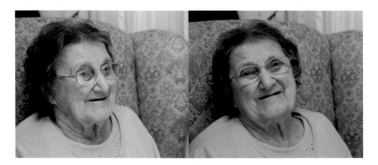

Balancing what is important to, with what is important for Nora

It is important to Nora that when she goes to bed, she can see the long mirror on her wardrobe. This allows her to see whether there are people in the corridor. This helps Nora feel safe and secure. Nora used to become upset and anxious when the night staff shut the door, which they did because the door was a fire door and regulations dictated that it had to be closed. Nora would sometimes struggle to get out of bed to open the door, only for night staff to close it again as they did their round.

Although what was important for Nora was being met, as she was safer from fire by having a fire door, this was not in balance with what is important to her. It is important to her to look out into the corridor.

Steve and Sheila (the owners) had a magnetic smoke detector fitted to the bottom of Nora's door. This means that Nora is still safe from fire (important for her) and has what is important to her, as the door stays open and she can look into the corridor. The detector cost £200, but it means that Nora can now sleep through the night, rather than being anxious that somebody may be out in the corridor.

Nora's story illustrates the importance of finding out what matters to and for someone, and finding a balance that works.

Gathering information and recording it on a one-page profile

A one-page profile is a way to record what people appreciate about someone, what matters to them (what is important to them) and what good support looks like (what is important for them). The staff supporting Alice started her one-page profile by finding out what a good day and a bad day looked like for her and we describe what they found opposite. Then we look at Mary's story, which explains how you can gather this information, through conversation or an informal 'one-page profile meeting'.[2]

Alice Peacock's good days and bad days

We all have good days and bad days. What amounts to a good day for you may equate to someone else's bad day. Your good day may start with listening to hip-hop music as you get up. For others, anything other than the soothing tones of classical music or catching up with the news would be the beginning of a bad day. Many older people (those in hospital, those attending or receiving services on a regular basis, and those who live in communal settings) have been subjected to other people's choice of morning music, with little thought about the impact of this.

One of the ways to develop a one-page profile is to start learning about a person's good days and their bad days. This can also lead to decisions and actions about how to help the person have more good days.

---

2   For information on One-page Profile Meetings see www.helensanderson associates.co.uk

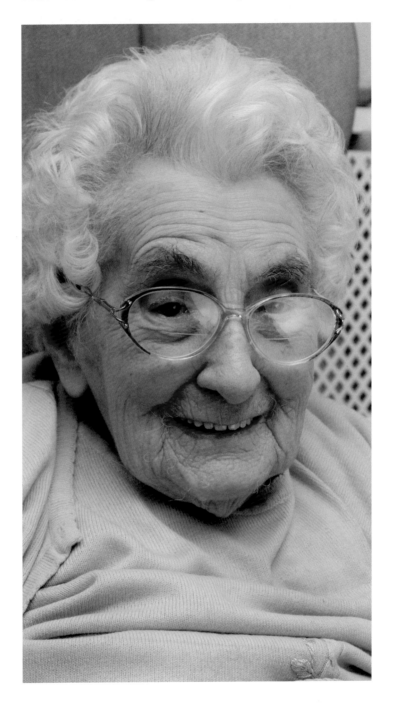

Alice has an ever-ready smile. She is a gentle woman who lives in a residential home. She never complains. This makes it more challenging to discover what a bad day looks like for her, so staff based their account on times when they have seen Alice looking sad or distressed. Here's their list of what makes a good day for Alice.

What makes a good day for Alice

- People taking the time to chat with her.

- Having visitors from church.

- Having flowers in a vase in her bedroom.

- Having chocolates with soft fillings to eat.

- Jim and Edith (her brother and his wife) visiting.

- June bringing the church newsletter and somebody sitting and reading through it with her.

- Going outside for a short walk if she wants to.

- A bath with bubbles.

What makes a bad day for Alice

- Feeling confused and worried when she believes her mother is waiting at home for her and she cannot get out of the front door.

- Being afraid her mother will be very vexed with her for not going home.

- Walking around the home in a state of confusion.

- Being hot, flushed and breathless.

- Nobody chatting to her.

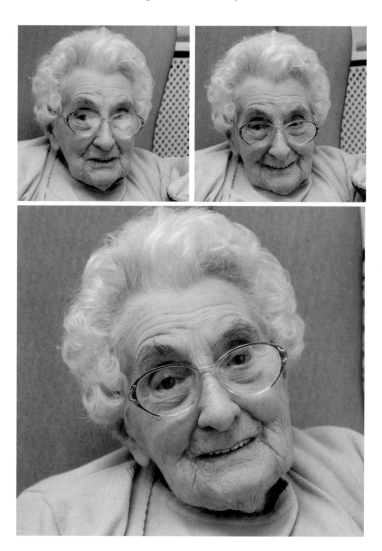

From this information, and from talking to Jim, Edith and June, the staff developed a list of what is important to Alice, and began her one-page profile.

Important to Alice

- Living in the Millbrook area (see Alice's graphic history in the history chapter). Her whole life centres around living in Millbrook.

- To have company and live with other people who like her. She will say: 'I'm all right here with the gang', meaning the other people who live at the home.

- To chat with staff and the other people who live there.

- To see June each month, and for June to bring her the church newsletter.

- To be able to go outside for a walk whenever she wants to.

- To see Jim and Edith every week.

- To hug people she cares about.

- To have fresh flowers in her bedroom all the time.

- To have soft-centred chocolates and sweets when she wants them.

- For staff to acknowledge Alice each time they pass by her.

- To have a bath with bubbles in and having water poured over her back at least three times a week.

The staff separated what matters to Alice from the best ways to support her. They included information that was not just about Alice's good and bad days, but also described what needs to happen to keep Alice healthy, safe and well.

How best to support Alice

- Ensure she wears her built-up slippers.

- Read the church newsletter with her; she struggles to read it alone. Share her enthusiasm and pleasure in hearing what is happening within the church community, as she was once at the heart of it.

- Always acknowledge Alice. She will beam at you and probably say, 'Eeh, well, fancy seeing you here.' She will then laugh. Have a chat with her, be interested in what she has to say. She will tell you so much about her life. Ask her to show you her history map – she will enjoy telling you her tales. Alice was a keen birdwatcher in the past; she may like talking about it.

- When Alice is having meat in her meals, it must be cooked until very tender.

- Alice struggles to eat fruit with skin on such as grapes, but enjoys bananas and tinned fruit.

- Alice will almost always say hello when you walk by her. Always acknowledge her, as she will forget that you have already said hello. When you are in the room and Alice says, 'Oy, oy, oy', she wants you to acknowledge her and have a chat.

- Be aware that Alice may be a little low once Jim and Edith leave after a visit.

- If Alice's glasses have slipped down her nose, ask her if she would like you to push them up for her.

Mary Hall

Mary was born and bred in Gorton in Manchester, a real Mancunian through-and-through, and she is described as 'salt of the earth'. She married Albert (her late husband), and they had four children: Brenda, Maureen, Brian and Karen. Mary is very close to her family, particularly Brenda, who visits often. During her life Mary was very much a family woman. She raised her children, and had various jobs working as a domestic.

Mary went to live in a care home in 2009. The organisation wanted to deliver more personalised support to everyone who lived at the care home, and started by introducing one-page profiles.

They did this through having informal 'one-page profile meetings' with the family and staff who knew the person well.

June, the manager of the home where Mary lives, asked Mary and her daughter Brenda if they could meet informally for an hour with her and Gill to develop Mary's one-page profile. They agreed and met in Mary's room, as this was where Mary felt most comfortable. They held the meeting mid-afternoon as Brenda said she always found her mum to be at her best at that time of the day. Gill led the conversation, gently asking a range of different questions. She asked about what good days and bad days were like; and what was working and not working for Mary from her perspective, from Benda's perspective and from June's perspective. She discovered what Brenda admired about her mum, and what June valued about Mary. Through these conversations Gill learned what was important to Mary, what good support looked like from her perspective, and what people appreciated about her.

Gill learned that what makes a good day for Mary is to have some chocolate. Her daughter Brenda said that there's always a supply in a cupboard in her bedroom so that staff can offer her chocolate every day.

Mary loves hugs and affection when she's in the mood, and she'll let you know when she's in the mood. She's a very direct woman. She loves to be complimented and enjoys conversation. She will tell you about the possessions she has in her room: the pictures of her family, her CDs, cushions and throws.

Having a sing-song is always good from Mary's perspective. She loves to watch the proms on television, or anything to do with royalty such as the changing of the guard.

For Mary bad days happen when she feels she's missing out on fun things that are going on in the home due to the amount of physical support that she needs.

As a result of learning and recording this information in Mary's one-page profile, staff were able to have good conversations with her by talking about things of interest to her such as her daughter Brenda, family life and the royal family. Her favourite music can always be heard playing when she is on bed rest and staff know to ensure her TV is on if any of her favourite programmes are on.

Asking different questions led to different conversations that led to a thorough understanding of what matters to Mary and how she wants to be supported. This is the information that all staff need to ensure a person's support is tailored to them, the very bedrock of personalisation.

One-page profiles

One-page profiles reflect what matters to someone and how they want to be supported – the balance between what is important to and for them. They are developed through conversation and this can start with talking about good days and bad days, or an informal meeting. One-page profiles begin with appreciations so that the person is valued for who they are, their characteristics and gifts.

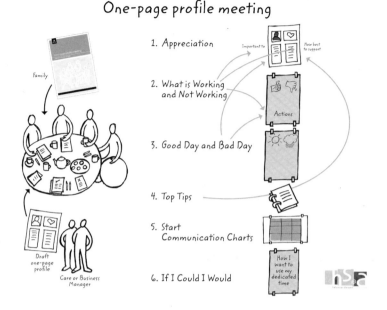

Figure 1.1 The one-page profile meeting

When and how one-page profiles can be useful

ASSESSMENTS

Knowing what is important to and how best to support an older person can help to keep an assessment focused on the person, their story, their view of their needs and what will help to meet them. A one-page profile can start as part of the assessment process and then be built on and developed over time. Staff find that as well as asking the required assessment questions, asking a few additional questions about good days and bad days, and what is working and not working, enables them to start a one-page profile at the same time as completing the assessment.

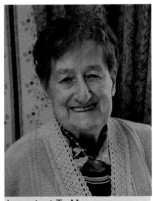

WHAT THOSE WHO KNOW MARY SAY THEY LIKE AND ADMIRE ABOUT HER

- She has a fantastic, cheeky sense of humour
- She is an eternal optimist
- Affectionate and loyal
- Very nurturing
- Sociable and caring
- Infectious giggle
- Very kind

Important To Mary

- Her niece Susan and sister Agnes visiting every Saturday.
- To entertain Susan and Agnes with tea and biscuits when they visit. Mary loves to set out a napkin on the table to serve it 'properly'
- To have a cake and tea party on her birthday and to invite her family.
- Mary enjoys taking new people moving in to Oakwood House under her wing, she will show them around and generally help them to settle in.
- On days when the hairdresser visits, Mary enjoys spending time with the people who live downstairs when they go upstairs to get their hair done, especially Margaret and Ann Hall.
- Being around people, she thrives in company and particularly enjoys visits from June and other lay preachers from church. She enjoys the hymns and communal prayers.
- That she follows her own routines which she has developed and structuring her day giving her a general sense of wellbeing.
- Going to her bedroom after lunch to read – romantic novels are favourite – and saying her prayers.
- Having her cup of tea and a glass of orange juice at 3.00pm, Mary loves a 'natter' with the member of staff who takes her afternoon drink up.

How best to Support Mary

- When you take Mary's cup of tea and orange juice into her room at 3.00pm, chat with her for a little while – this is the time she will share any anxieties or worries or off load some small frustrations she may have.
- Mary does not like any meals with minced beef or fish and when this is on the menu she must be offered an alternative.
- If paste or any fish is on the teatime sandwich Mary must be offered alternatives such as jam, banana or cheese.
- Mary always has a tray of tea taken up for Susan, Agnes and herself when they visit. Mary keeps the biscuits in her bedroom.
- Due to Mary's willingness to help new residents settle in they occasionally rely on her too much and she may need some support in separating herself from this.
- Mary doesn't enjoy spending time in the downstairs lounge.
- Mary will stick to her own routines e.g. washing in a certain way, applying cream and wearing only 2 outfits out of a large wardrobe – never pass comment or criticise Mary on this.
- Mary would dress in one of her 'best outfits' if something was happening that she would see as a special occasion such as the entertainer coming in, if she was going out or there was a party at the home.
- Mary must have her underwear back from the laundry as soon as possible otherwise she will worry about this.
- Mary derives much comfort from her routines, ensure you follow her preferred bedtime routine she has developed for support staff to follow.
- Mary laughs easily when amused and cries openly when upset, if Mary is angry she will be unusually quiet – once you pick up that she is quiet and sit down and talk to her she will tell you what has happened to anger her.

Figure 1.2 Mary's one-page profile

CARE AND SUPPORT PLANNING

Having a record of what is important to and important for someone makes it much easier to translate the outcomes of an assessment into clear and personalised support plans and to organise other care arrangements. It can also be a good way of checking back with the person that what is recorded and what is set out in a care and support plan makes sense to them, and matches their understanding of what has been agreed or identified in a plan. Some organisations include a one-page profile at the beginning of the care plan.

FIRST CONTACT WITH A SERVICE

As these stories show, one-page profiles can make a huge difference to older people and their families, and to staff in getting to know someone and understand who they are – rather than just seeing an older person as a set of needs or problems. Developing or building on a one-page profile can help to build trust and confidence in the service for the older person and their family. It sends a very strong message that this person is important, that staff care about them, and that knowing them matters to us.

MOVING TO A NEW PLACE

If an older person is moving to a new kind of domestic arrangement – for example, to supported or warden-assisted housing or a care home – developing and sharing one-page profiles can be a practical and insightful way of finding out what's important about and to an older person as the first step in building new relationships and friendships.

REVIEWS

Knowing what matters to the person, and what good support looks like, provides a place to start when you review the service that they are receiving. Reviews are also an opportunity to update the one-page profile.

DAY-TO-DAY LIFE

Where someone receives services and support from a range of services or professionals, sharing a one-page profile is a way to make sure that the person does not have to repeat information, and that all services are able to provide consistent support.

Daytime support or care homes often have a programme of activities that older people can join. One-page profiles provide all the information you need to help design a programme that reflects people's individual interests. One care home, for example, looked at the one-page profiles of everyone they supported to find the top ten interests and based their activities programme on this, with a dramatic improvement in people's enjoyment of and participation in the activities.

Chapter 2
Relationship Circles

Relationships are everything. As Paul Tournier says:

> It is impossible to over-emphasise the immense need people have to be really listened to, to be taken seriously, to be understood. No one can develop freely in this world and find a full life, without feeling understood by at least one person.[1]

For almost all of us, thinking about what matters to us will include people and relationships. We now know that being lonely has the same impact on health as smoking 15 cigarettes a day. Paying attention to relationships is essential for health and wellbeing, yet they are rarely seen as a priority for services.

A relationship map or circle is a good way of identifying and capturing who is important to an older person, to ensure that there is 'at least one person' and to actively seek to widen the connections and relationships that someone has. A relationship circle or map lets us learn more about the people in someone's life, both who they are, and the depth of the relationships. It can quickly provide a picture of how connected someone is, or if they are lonely, and the balance between family, friends and staff in their life.

There are different ways that relationship circles and maps can be represented. One common approach was developed by Judith Snow and uses concentric circles to represent the closeness of relationships. The following is an adapted version.

---

1   Townier, P. (1967) *To Understand Each Other.* Louisville, KY: John Knox Press.

In this relationship circle the people placed in the closest ring would be those whom the person loves; the second ring would contain people the person likes; the third ring would be people the person knows, and people who are paid to be in that person's life, like support staff, professionals or hairdressers.

Relationships

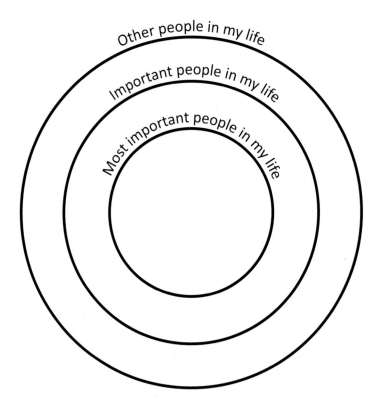

Figure 2.1: A relationship circle

Thinking about relationships and recording them on a relationship map can lead to questions and actions, for example:

- If the person does not have many people in their life, or their map or circle contains mainly staff, then ask 'What would it take to increase the number and depth of your relationships?'

- If the person has recently moved, then ask 'Who would you like to stay connected to and what can we do to help that?'

- If the person needs support to stay connected to family and friends, then ask 'How can we support you to stay in touch, for example, through cards, phone calls and visits?'

Jakob had moved and knew no-one, and Audrey was recently bereaved and lonely. For both, doing a relationship circle was a way to start thinking about how they could meet new people and increase the relationships in their life

Jakob Kravits

Jakob is 78 and lives in a council flat in Portsmouth, but is originally from Ukraine. He was a refugee in Germany before moving to the UK in the 1970s. English is his third language. His marriage to an English woman broke down many years ago, and it seems their child had died.

When we first met Jakob he didn't know anyone in Portsmouth and had no living relatives. Although he was not eligible for any social care service, he had been ringing the duty social work number several times a week, in great distress.

Jakob was very reluctant to leave his flat and was generally very anxious and unhappy. He talked about going to Leicester, where he lived with his ex-wife, even though he did not know anyone who lived there. When social workers had visited him (following his calls) he had not wanted to pursue anything that they suggested in the way of local support, such as the social services funded shopping service (to help him think about taking care of himself and eating well) or the local Good

Neighbours scheme (a volunteer-run befriending scheme). Other than ringing the duty social work number, Jakob's only other contact was with his Tenancy Support Worker. Using an adapted relationship circle helped Jakob to discover that he really wanted to meet people and make friends. He was lonely, isolated and very unhappy.

Jakob's Tenancy Support Worker, Julie, helped him to think about his relationships.

She was already involved in his life as she was helping him to sort out some rent arrears and benefits claims. Julie's role was flexible and she talked to Jakob about using person-centred thinking tools together to think about relationships, and what Jakob wanted in his life. They developed a plan to try to increase the number of people in his life by expanding what he was doing, and joining clubs.

Jakob's life changed a lot over the next few months. He significantly expanded the number of people in his relationship circle. Equally importantly, though he was extremely reluctant beforehand to try anything, he began to try all sorts of things of his own volition.

Soon Jakob:

- was going regularly to a new, monthly Age Concern 'Gentleman's Club', getting there on his own, on public transport

- was playing chess with a man he met there who shares his love of the game

- had visited the local D-Day museum with his new friend

- had attended a local voluntary organisation's Christmas lunch, where he met more people whom he wants to see again

- had offered to teach another man chess in return for computer lessons.

He soon no longer needed to see Julie because her role of Tenancy Support Worker, with its associated tasks, was fulfilled. Jakob no longer calls the duty social work team and no longer seems worried about or interested in revisiting Leicester.

Audrey Peters

Audrey, 73, had been widowed for 18 months when we first got to know her. Her daughter, who lived some distance away, was very worried that her mum had lost her previous outgoing personality and sociability. Audrey and her husband had not long moved to Portsmouth (from South Wales) when he died.

At the beginning, Audrey told us that some days she would get on any of the buses that stopped at the end of her road, and just stay on it in the hope that she would find someone to have a chat with that day.

Audrey worked with a Circles facilitator for five hours of visits. They began by developing Audrey's relationship circle. They had a focus for each visit or meeting that they held. Audrey particularly enjoyed being set a small task to report back on at the next meeting. Over five visits, these tasks included: completing the mapping of her own circle; going to a local computer club for which her facilitator had found details; and going to the local Methodist church and collecting a copy of their newsletter and details of services.

This approach seemed to help Audrey by enabling her to take several small steps that led cumulatively to large changes in her life. It also helped her facilitator to plan each visit, to start the conversation each time, and to make sure progress on Audrey's goals and wishes was kept on track.

By the end of these sessions Audrey told us she had:

- joined a club

- made five new friends

- gone out twice to the theatre with some of these new friends

- found and employed a regular gardener

- enjoyed a new craft session at the club and continued with it at home

- become much closer to her daughters, brother and sister-in-law

- made plans for a trip to the USA to see her Canadian-based daughter

- plans to find a Methodist church to worship at again

- plans to learn to use a computer

- plans to become a 'Good Neighbours' volunteer.

By the time her facilitator finished these five sessions their friendship and regard for each other was growing. They hoped to stay in contact even when the work relationship was over, and had already enjoyed a theatre trip together. Audrey's circle has grown significantly. She has now added the following people to her relationship circle:

- a friendship with the local Mr KleenEzey

- the gardener

- her facilitator.

Audrey also importantly identified that some of her existing (not close) relationships had changed. She had felt able to tell her brother and sister-in-law and her two daughters something from her past that she had kept secret for a long time. She told her facilitator that she felt much closer to those people as a result.

Audrey felt that the changes in her life were all down to the facilitator; but the facilitator was equally clear that nothing would have changed had Audrey not been willing to try and to do as much as she had.

When can relationship circles be useful?

Relationship circles provide a starting place for thinking about who matters to someone, and what this means for their life and support. It can help them to think about how they may want to reconnect with people from their past, and the support they need to stay in touch with people or develop new relationships.

ASSESSMENTS

Knowing what is important to someone will include the people in their life. Doing a relationship circle at assessment can be a way to explore who the person is connected to, and this could influence decisions about where the person may want to live, or who may want to provide informal support.

If the person does not use words to communicate, completing a relationship circle with the person who knows them best will be vital to know who has the information needed to complete any assessment or care and support plan.

CARE AND SUPPORT PLANNING

Knowledge of family, friends and neighbours should have an impact not just on what support services focus on, but how support is delivered. Supporting people to stay connected to family and friends will have a long-term beneficial impact on people's health. The process called 'Just Enough Support'[2] involves making sure that we think creatively about the support that someone needs, and fully consider support from friends

---

2   A process for looking at the support a person needs and how this can be creatively delivered. See www.helensandersonassociates.co.uk for more information.

and family, assistive technology and community assets, as well as paid support.

MOVING TO A NEW PLACE

If an older person is moving to a new place, it is very important to pay attention to the connections and relationships that the person wants to keep. Doing a relationship circle is a way to start that conversation, and to think about support to develop new relationships as well.

REVIEWS

A relationship circle is a way to talk about who to invite to the person's review. Looking at what is working and not working about relationships is important to cover in a person-centred review, given the importance of relationships to health and wellbeing.

Chapter 3
Communication

Older people must have the power to communicate and to be understood if they are to have choice and control in their life – in fact, to have any quality of life at all. It is easy to assume that older people who cannot talk have little to say. Nora, whom we met in the previous chapter, can only say 'yes', yet has at least four different ways of saying it, each conveying a different meaning. She has plenty to communicate, if we can also listen to the subtleties of her expression and body language.

When many staff members support someone, each of them may have a different idea of what the person is communicating with their behaviours or words.

The communication chart is a powerful and simple way to record how an older person communicates (see Figure 3.1 on page 60). This is critical to someone who doesn't talk, and is also important where people use only a few words, or communicate most powerfully with their behaviours.

The communication chart has four headings:

1. *What is happening* describes the circumstances.

2. *What the person does* clearly describes what the person says or does in enough detail that someone reading the chart who has not seen this behaviour would still recognise it. Where a communication is hard to describe (e.g. a facial expression) you could use a picture. Some people have even developed video communication charts.

3. *We think it means* describes the meaning that people think is present – a best guess. It is not uncommon for there to be more than one meaning for a single behaviour. Where this is the case, all of the meanings should be listed.

4. *We should* describes what staff should do to respond to what the person is saying with their behaviour. This section gives us an insight into how the older person is perceived and supported.

It's easiest to complete a communication chart by starting with the two inside columns (starting with 'What the person does', and moving onto 'We think it means'). Following this, work out to the two outside columns ('What is happening' and 'We should').

As an example, Nora's communication chart is below.

When people don't communicate with many or any words, starting with a communication chart is crucial. There can be no choice or control in someone's life if we do not know how to communicate with them.

When can communication charts be useful?

ASSESSMENTS

Of all the person-centred thinking tools that could ideally be started in assessment, communication charts and one-page profiles are the most important. If assessment is the access point to services, it must begin with a clear understanding of exactly how the older person communicates if they are to have any choice or control over their life or services.

CARE AND SUPPORT PLANNING

Any care and support planning needs to include how the person communicates. The older person cannot be involved in the care and support planning process without this information.

FIRST CONTACT WITH A SERVICE

To enable staff and professionals to get to know someone quickly and develop a relationship requires that they know how the person communicates, what good support looks like and what matters to the person. Therefore making sure that communication charts and one-page profiles are in place should be a priority for any service as it welcomes new people. If these are in place and used consistently, staff can build relationships and trust from the beginning.

In an emergency – for example, an admission to hospital – a communication chart can make all the difference to the patient's experience and how well nurses are able to care for them.

REVIEWS

Where people do not use words to speak this does not mean that they cannot be present and involved in their reviews. Communication charts help staff know the best ways to involve people in preparing for their review, and contributing to it.

Reviews are also an opportunity to update communication charts and one-page profiles.

What is happening where/when	When Nora does this	We think it means	And we should
Anytime	Nora shouts 'yes'	She wants to go to the bathroom	Support her to go to the bathroom
Nora is being asked to make a choice or answer a question, for example, choosing her own clothes	Nora says 'yes' but her facial expression is cross and her tone is sharp	She doesn't like the item of clothing you are showing her or the answer to the question is no	Respect the answer to the question is no. Show her more options when choosing her clothes
Nora is being asked to make a choice or answer a question	Nora smiles and says 'yes' enthusiastically	Nora is telling us 'yes'	Depends on the question or choice but respond accordingly, letting Nora know we understand she has told us 'yes'
In the evening	Nora will take her feet off her footstool, remove the rug from her knee and look in an obvious way at the clock	She wants to get up out of her armchair and go to bed – usually 7.30ish	Check with Nora if she wants to go to bed. If so, support her (see Nora's going to bed routine)
Anytime	Nora grimaces and says 'yes' in a cross tone or swears	She is unhappy – perhaps her routine has not run like clockwork, the nurse is late or early (Nora hasn't finished her breakfast), somebody may have gone in her bedroom or she doesn't like what is on TV	Sit and talk to her
Anytime	Nora holds your hand/ smiles at everybody	She is happy	Enjoy her company

Figure 3.1: Nora's communication chart

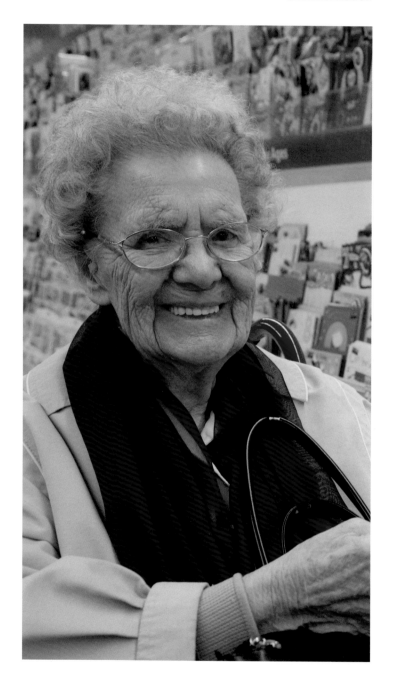

Chapter 4
Histories

Our histories make us what we are. Older people's histories can easily become lost or be left untold. A conscious effort to listen to and record individual histories can help staff to understand and appreciate people in a different way, and in doing so develop different relationships with them. This can also happen within families – especially between different generations.

There are many ways to capture and record histories – for example, with photographs, family trees and scrapbooks, through miniature histories in objects, with graphics or simply by writing them. Websites and commercially available packages can help to capture family histories, and most families would be delighted to help. Histories, or life stories, are used extensively with people living with dementia, usually as part of a care and support plan. In this chapter we share the difference that this approach can make, and the benefits of doing this visually, so that people can refer to it.

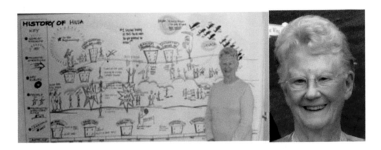

Hilda Williams

Hilda is an inspirational woman who is proud to be 93 and living in her own home in Blackpool. You would only need to spend a brief amount of time with her to feel the joy for life she exudes.

A film buff, her knowledge of the movies right back to the 1930s is incredible. She has travelled widely to visit her daughter Joan and her family, as their work has meant they have lived in many different countries. Her latest holiday photos are from Hollywood.

Hilda was talking with her great-niece, Babs, about how the world has changed and about her hopes and fears around getting older. What really frightened her was that her memory wasn't as good as it used to be and that:

> Some day I may not remember what a great life I have lived so far.

Babs and Hilda decided to spend a few hours together to capture Hilda's life on a graphic history map. This was the start, and now they are scanning in family photos to create a family history book as well.

Alice Peacock

Alice used to work in the residential home where she now lives. The imposing house, Millbrook, used to belong to a mill owner, and Alice was the nanny to his children. Once the children had grown, she became the housekeeper and cook. She was a well-known local character, always at the heart of St. James' Church community. She is great company and has always loved to chat with other people, showing a real interest in what they have to say. Alice is delighted when staff, visitors and the people she lives with at the home chat with her, and she loves to be acknowledged as people walk by, even if that means saying hello a number of times, as Alice will forget that you have already spoken to her.

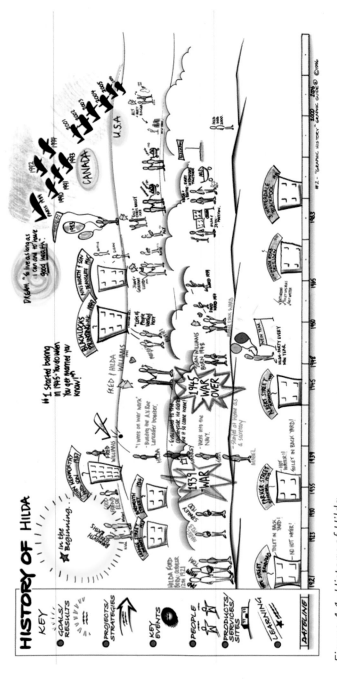

Figure 4.1: History of Hilda

The staff and a volunteer who enjoys drawing worked with Alice to create a picture of her past (a graphic history) and some of what is important to her. It's up on the wall now to give people clues about Alice's past, so that they can talk with her and ask her about it.

'It brightens my day to have people sit and ask me about my picture. I love talking about Millbrook and telling my many tales,' says Alice.

We knew so little of this information – especially about Alice's past. Who would have thought Alice was a keen birdwatcher and rambler? She has lived here almost six years, and all that time we didn't know. I've learnt so much about her by using this approach. It's just brilliant. (A staff member).

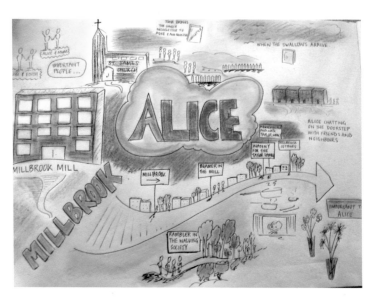

Figure 4.2: Alice's history graphic

Hilda and her family wanted to record her history, so that they could talk about it and remind Hilda of the great life she had lived. Alice's history gave staff a new perspective on who she was, with increased understanding and respect, and again, gave people a way to start conversations.

Recording histories, or life story work, is enjoyable for the person, family and staff, and can enhance self-worth and wellbeing.

When can recording histories be useful?

ASSESSMENT

Through the process of assessment, information about the person's past may naturally emerge. Making sure that this is recorded can ensure that information is not lost, and can be built on and expanded later, when creating a life story or picture.

CARE AND SUPPORT PLANNING

Many care homes have a section in their planning paperwork to record the person's history. These enable the person to be seen in the context of their history, before learning about what matters to them now, through developing their one-page profile. Knowing about a person's history can sometimes help develop outcomes and goals for how they want to live now. For example, the history may give clues about past hobbies and interests that the person may want to explore again. Knowing what has worked and not worked for someone in the past is important as it informs how they are supported now.

FIRST CONTACT WITH A NEW SERVICE

Knowing someone's history, as well as what is important to them now, is a powerful and effective way to develop relationships with new staff. This ensures that the person is seen as an individual, and recognised for what they have experienced or achieved in their life.

Moving to a care home or other form of supported accommodation can be a traumatic experience for many different reasons. Histories can help staff and others working in or visiting that home to get to know someone well. Having framed photos, pictures, framed family trees or other ways of representing history like the history frame in Figure 4.3 are great ways to personalise people's living areas. People can use them to introduce themselves to new members of staff or volunteers.

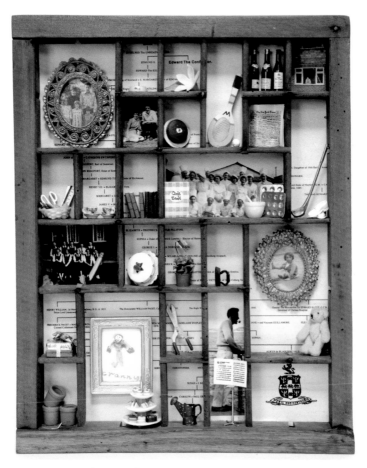

Figure 4.3: A history frame

Chapter 5

Wishing

What do you wish for? Is this any different to what older people wish for? In South Oxfordshire we asked a number of older people about their wishes and dreams as part of the Circles work described in the introduction.[1] We talked to people in group settings (day care centres, lunch clubs and social clubs) and asked what they wished for and what they thought it would take to make it happen. We did this because we wanted to find different ways in which interested organisations and individuals could think together about how to support people to work towards wishes, goals or dreams.

A session on wishes

Facilitators from the Older People's Programme ran a session with each group on wishes, and then kept in touch with the club organisers afterwards to give them some support and ideas to carry the work forward. There were between 15 and 20 people at each session. Many had disabilities and long-term conditions (including severe arthritis, Parkinson's disease, depression, a dementia or sensory impairment), which both they and others involved in their support assumed had stopped them from dreaming or pursuing their wishes. Others felt it was 'just their age'.

Our conversations about wishes revealed a different picture.

---

1   The Oxford circles and wishes project was run by the Older People's Programme with Age Concern Oxfordshire.

The wishes we were told

Overall, we asked around 80 older people about their wishes, from five different clubs and groups. Only a few people had no wish that they wanted to share with us. Of these, two could not think of anything because:

My time is full doing different things – I'm fully occupied.

My days are full with committee meetings, line dancing, bowls and Friday Club – weekends my family visit.

But most people had two or three wishes they could think of straight away. Some people needed a bit more of a chat before thinking of something – whether with us, or with another club member, or the club organiser or volunteers.

The wishes we were told are grouped under 11 general headings. This list of wishes includes those shared by the team as well as any shared by the clubs' staff and volunteers. We've included these wishes because, whilst we know which is which, we think that only some of these stand out as being obviously the wishes of younger or older people.

Interestingly, although some wishes might cost some money to achieve, only two people talked specifically about goods they wished they owned, or could buy:

I'd like a pair of amber earrings.

Find Cadbury's Old Jamaican chocolate bar, as I can't buy this in the shops any more.

Our reactions

Our reactions to older people's wishes are critical. We wondered whether many of us are too quick to write off an older person's wish, because:

- We are worried about the risks involved (sometimes without understanding what's involved at all!).

- It's not what we'd do.

- We'd love it to happen as well – but life isn't fair so why expect to have this?

- We dismiss it because we've heard it all before.

- We don't think that's what that older person should be doing.

Here are some examples

We held a sounding board seminar and invited a small number of key people nationally, who are interested in improving services for older people and in person-centred approaches. When we mentioned that lots of people had the wish to go in a hot-air balloon, one person said, 'Not that old chestnut again.'

At the same seminar, although we'd talked about a wide range of wishes (including the people who were looking into Voluntary Services Overseas, as they wanted to do voluntary work abroad), another person lamented about how limited older people's ambitions and goals are. At one of our Advisory Group meetings, we also heard this same view.

There is no doubt that we did not hear every single wish held by all the older people we met. But the ones we heard were genuinely held. If these are old chestnuts, or they fall short of the sorts of dreams and ambitions we believe we have for ourselves, we shouldn't let our disappointment cloud our responses to their dreams. In other words, it might well be an old chestnut – but it's their old chestnut, and that's what matters.

Setting up false expectations

One issue that we heard a lot from people across the sites was in essence an objection to asking the question at all. It can be paraphrased as:

You shouldn't ask because if you know you can't deliver, you've given someone false hope by setting up their expectations.

This seemed to be based on an assumption that we think we must fulfil everything we ask about. This belief seems to us to be fundamentally tied up with the last decades of social care practice, since the community care reforms of 1993. We are used now to the idea that there are limited funds and therefore limited opportunities. We are well versed in applying eligibility criteria, and in telling people they don't qualify for support.

Why have we come to assume that we have to fulfil everything for an older person – and so avoid asking about any aspect of life we can't arrange? If your friend says they want to go on a world cruise next year it's highly unlikely you'll rush out to raise the money to pay for it, organise their health jabs, pack their swimsuit, present them with the tickets and physically escort them on board.

But there's every chance you'll show a great interest in their plans, ask them how arrangements are going, keep an eye out for articles and bits of information that might be of help or interest to them, ask them to send you a postcard, and then look at their photographs and home video/DVD on their return. This approach is about doing a little bit of both – a bit of practical help, and a bit of encouragement and interest. How much of each will vary from person to person, and from situation to situation. But this is not the equivalent of you paying for and sorting out every aspect of your friend's cruise.

There is another important aspect to this. As you're not expected to deliver the whole wish, try not to take over. This approach isn't about helping you feel better because you 'did' something (in other words, you sorted it all out), it's about supporting someone else to play as big a part as they can in achieving their wish, in part because:

- that's what treating an adult like an adult means

- if the person can be encouraged by their own efforts, they may begin to tackle more for themselves.

Wherever possible, you should avoid creating a dependency on you to sort everything out. This means saying 'well done', just as you would to anyone you know who is doing something that might be difficult for them.

This is also why this is an approach and not a service.

Achieving the wishes

Some people, when asked, already had the contacts they needed to make their wish come true, but they weren't doing anything about it. What seemed to help them was talking to someone who took an interest and encouraged them.

In each case, the only question we had asked to start this part of the conversation going was:

- What would you need to do to make this happen?

Molly James – a visit to the Philippines

A good example was a woman whose wish was to go to the Philippines with her family. She had enough savings for a flight and her Philippina daughter-in-law went every year to stay with her own family and took her children. They were always inviting her to go too, so there would be no accommodation costs. She said:

> I've been saying for ages I'll do it, but that's definite. I'm going to ring my daughter-in-law tonight and tell her 'Book the tickets straight away and count me in'.

Vera Barnham – a horse event

A woman who used to go horse racing with her husband said she would like to go again. Her son had a share in a race horse so she would ask her family if they would take her to see it race, or take her to see her granddaughter at a gymkhana.

Janet Barnes – a hot-air balloon

One of the (several) people who wanted to go on a hot-air balloon ride had already been on one before, organised by her son. She decided to ask him if she could go again, as:

They're always asking me what I'd like for my birthday and Christmas, and I can never think of anything to ask for. If it's a lot of money maybe they could all chip in, or it could be my present for both. I don't need any more talc, that's for sure!

She said it wouldn't have occurred to her to ask for something like that if we hadn't been asking the question about wishes that day.

Tom Mills – going on a cruise

One person who wanted to take a cruise to visit about three different countries, wrote:

I am selling my house this year so feel this may well come true.

Of course, not everyone has the money or family to help achieve his or her wishes. Nor does everyone feel well enough to do precisely what he or she might like.

An African Safari trip

A man with a mild form of dementia said his wish was to go to see the Masai Mara, but he didn't think he was well enough to travel that far. Later that day, he came up with his own solution: he would like a day out at Longleat Safari Park, because his wish is to see African animals in the open.

Tony Roberts – in touch with nature again

A retired gamekeeper and a keen walker in the past, Tony is now 90 and said he would like to follow a particular local walk through a nature reserve. The club's deputy manager already knew the current gamekeeper of the estate through which most of the walk passes. She asked the gamekeeper about the possibility of using his Land Rover to take Tony along the route and he said he would be delighted to help. She gave the gamekeeper's telephone number to Tony, who was happy to make the call as this meant he could arrange the trip to suit him. Separately, she heard that Tony's daughter also knows he is to phone, so two of the people in his circle (or network) have been taking an interest and encouraging him to make the call, and are awaiting news that he has completed the walk.

When wishes aren't achieved

Some people may not be willing or able to achieve their wishes. One woman we met said she would love to have a massage and learn to swim, but she 'didn't have the guts'. She found ordinary life hard enough without adding something extra that she felt sure would make her more anxious. But she liked the idea of the wishes.

Another woman said she would love to get all her family together but, as this would mean 17 people, she didn't feel she would cope. She was adamant that no one was to mention this to her family, as she knew they would then sort it out and that, although she loved the idea, she would hate the reality. She said she wanted it to stay as her daydream.

A third woman told an interesting variation: the minute she mentioned to her daughter that she'd like to do something, it was organised for her – a trip to Dublin and an afternoon tea at a posh hotel were two recent examples. As a result, she was careful not to mention (even in passing) that there was something she would like to do: she loves these events, but thinks her daughter does too much for her and doesn't want to add to this if she can avoid it.

We shouldn't let the fact that something might not work out stop us trying things. Life really is like that sometimes. In your own life what do you do when something doesn't work out? Do you really stop trying anything ever again? When something doesn't work out for somebody you support, be clear whether you were the stumbling block and, if you were, either find someone else who will be able to support the person better than you did, or change your approach and ask the person if you might try again. If it doesn't work but there's nothing that could have been done to make it possible, try not to write off the whole approach.

Older people's top tips

At two of the clubs, we asked those present for their top tips for other older people on how to achieve their wishes. They said you need:

- enough money

- enough confidence

- to tell someone who might be able to help

- to ask someone else – would they like to do it too? Work on it together – or do they know someone else?

- to find out different or new ways of doing something or other ways of going about things.

On the money front, they had some additional tips:

- Ask your family (or whoever else buys you presents) if something could be for Christmas or birthday or both.

- Think of an alternative that would cost less.

- Team up with others so you can share and spread the costs.

- Save up, and look for discounts.

Check your own assumptions: does your age really get in the way of you doing something? Make sure you find out before reaching your decision. Many people had told us that they didn't want or need to explore other aspects of person-centred planning, but they were keen to share and explore their own personal goals and dreams – their wishes.

Summary of how wishes and wishing can be used

Asking someone about their wishes, and/or listening carefully to what they say in general conversation (which might reveal these wishes) can:

- Help to personalise the support that someone receives in small but vitally important ways. Often what people share are not big things, but important ways of doing things, past interests and friendships that they want to renew, or skills they want to develop. If costs are involved, they may well be personal expenses, and this can help to identify the priorities that person wants to focus on in order to have a good quality of life (e.g., paying for a taxi to go and visit a friend, or arranging a lift with someone else).

- Help to enrich someone's life and increase their control over what happens on a daily or weekly basis – moving their experience from one of surviving to thriving in a relatively short space of time. This can be especially important if someone is living in a communal setting such as a care home or other supported accommodation, where everything is organised for them and they therefore have little control over day-to-day decisions.

- Identify shared interests between two or more people – and therefore forge new friendships and networks. This can be particularly important if someone's network has diminished over time, or suddenly.

- Be part of a strategy for coping or living with depression or increasing low mood, through finding the things that brighten someone's day, or motivate them to get out and about and do the things they used to do, or always wanted to do.

- Help with decision making and building confidence in problem-solving by making wishes happen by working with others, or on their own.

Wishes in a care home

One care home is paying attention to wishes in a different way. They are talking to each person about what they would like to do if they could, thinking together about 'If I could, I would…'

Each person has two hours a month of support from a staff member of their choice, to help them achieve their wish.[2]

Summary

In all of this, it's important to remember that if we don't ask, we may never hear about someone else's wishes. We might not ask if we are worried that the person will think we are going to make their wishes come true for them and we don't want to have to do this or don't have time or other resources at hand. We often forget to think of who else might be able to help – including the person themselves. It may not occur to us to ask. The way we ask is also important, as is the way we respond to what we're told.

---

2   For more information on this, see the book about Bruce Lodge, *Making Individual Service Funds Work For People with Dementia Living in Care Homes*, (2014) published by Jessica Kingsley Publishers.

We also need to pay attention to what someone says in general conversation, and how we're being told something. You may be being told a wish. If you are the one person who will ever hear this wish – and you may only be told once – then if you miss it, the wish may never surface again.

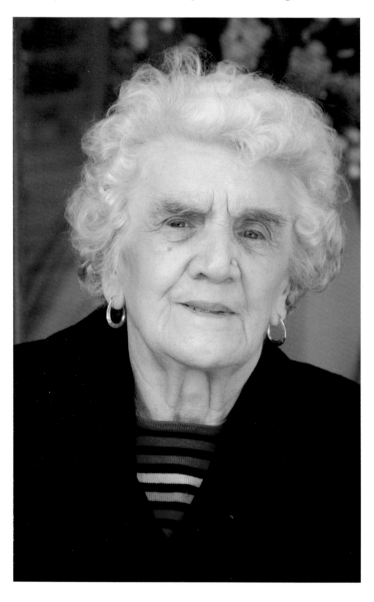

Chapter 6

Working and Not Working

For each of us, there are areas of our life that are working well and areas that are not working which we would like to change. Simply finding out from an older person about what is working and not working in their life tells us so much. This information may be used to change what can be changed, make sure that what is working continues and help us to understand what really matters to people.

Finding out what is working and not working is most powerful when it is considered from different perspectives, for example, those of the person and their family or staff. This is what happens in a person-centred review.

Beatrice Kelly

Beatrice broke her hip in a fall on some ice 15 years ago. This forced her to leave her home and she now lives in a care home.

She is dignified and elegant and was a successful career woman. A former head teacher, she later worked within Salford's education department, overseeing standards in all secondary schools in the authority.

Beatrice will talk about the great sense of loss she feels at no longer being involved with the community and how she misses having her own front door. She hates the locked doors at the care home that stop her getting out. She finds the temperature in the home too high, which makes her feel uncomfortable. She also struggles with having to eat at set times and feels this inflexibility is unjust.

Beatrice talks of her frustration at not being able to get around easily. She hates the Zimmer frame and, due to health and safety regulations, staff are not allowed to let Beatrice link arms with them for support. She would love to walk down to the library, a short walk from the home, but has to rely on the mobile service, which she occasionally misses if she is having an afternoon nap when it calls. She spends a lot of time knitting: she has always enjoyed knitting her own clothes but rarely has the opportunity to get out shopping for patterns. Beatrice says:

I was one hell of a shopper in my day, but don't get a chance any more. I miss my country walks, too. I was a great rambler.

Although Beatrice says she has come to terms with having to move out of her own beautiful house to live in the care home, she says:

After all these years, I still really miss being able to shut my front door, close the curtains and settle down for the evening to do as I please.

She does, however, have things she enjoys at the care home. She enjoys sitting in her room at the home in the evenings and reading her newspaper or watching TV – especially *Coronation Street* and *Emmerdale*. Beatrice enjoys reading and Bernard Cornwell is her favourite author, although she says, 'I'll read just about any fiction.'

Important To Beatrice

To be called Beatrice, not Beattie.

To choose when I eat. I like my tea around 6pm, not 4.30pm, and that I watch TV whilst I eat.

To read in bed for an hour before sleeping – any crime fiction is my favourite.

To have my cotton blouses starched and ironed.

Watching my soap operas. Coronation Street and Emmerdale are my favourites.

I love knitting my own clothes.

My photograph albums of my son George growing up and late husband Ben.

To chat with people about my life, especially my last job before retiring, when I was an Education Inspector.

I must go out once a week shopping. I especially enjoy choosing my own knitting patterns.

To have my morning newspaper every day, the Mail and Mail on Sunday are my favourites.

I love walking – anywhere these days, but where there are fields is my favourite.

To feel fresh and not over heated.

To wear my own clothes. I must not be dressed in other people's clothes. I hate this!

What those who know Beatrice say they like and admire about her

Always has a kind word for everybody.

A strong and gentle woman.

Great integrity.

The gentle way she sits and talks with me.

Her determination.

How best to support Beatrice

That only people I know well help me in the toilet and bathroom.

Recognise my embarrassment at needing help in the bathroom and toilet; be sensitive & kind with me.

Don't leave me on the toilet a long time. Wait at the door so I can call you when I am ready.

Let me link you when I walk; I hate the zimmer.

Heat my meals when I want them; don't tell me when I must eat.

I like lots of cups of tea – not just at set times. Please make me one when I ask.

Let me know if the mobile library service calls. If I am having a snooze, I miss them.

Beatrice

Figure 6.1: Beatrice's one-page profile

A great frustration for Beatrice is that she is unable to wash her own clothes and, in her view, the home's laundry service leaves a lot to be desired. She also struggles with the amount of support she requires to look after herself physically. Beatrice feels terribly undermined when staff members she doesn't know turn up on shift and support her to use the toilet, and with bathing, dressing and undressing.

'I feel defeated, it feels like nobody's listening when I tell staff how unhappy I am about this.' Beatrice asks herself, 'What have I come to when a stranger is putting me on the toilet?'

Even worse for Beatrice is when some staff do not wait at the door while she uses the toilet, but go away and do something else.

Then they come back to take me off the toilet when it suits them.

Sally, a new senior staff member, helped Beatrice to summarise what was working and not working for her. Sally also talked with staff, and captured what was working and not working from their perspectives. This is what she found.

What is working for Beatrice

- Reading her books at bedtime and having a variety to choose from.

- Watching the TV and never missing her soaps.

- Knitting.

- Having a daily newspaper delivered.

What is not working for Beatrice

- Not being able to go out for walks (has only been out twice in the last three months to buy her patterns).

- Not having someone to link her arm to support her for the ten-minute walk up to the library.

- Using the Zimmer frame to walk.

- Having to eat meals at set times, with no flexibility each day.

- Staff calling her Beattie.

- That her family do not visit her.

- Her blouses not being starched.

- Always being too hot.

- Not being able to open windows.

- Having other people's clothes put on her and other people wearing her clothes.

- Having name tags on her clothes.

- Clothes being spoiled in the laundry.

What is working for the staff team

- People's clothes being clearly name tagged.

- Beatrice eating at the same time as everybody else.

- Beatrice walking with her Zimmer frame for support.

- Beatrice enjoying her books and TV programmes.

- Beatrice fitting in most of the time by eating her meals with other residents.

- The mobile library service.

- Catching up on other jobs once Beatrice has been positioned on the toilet.

- Keeping the home warm for all the residents.

- Keeping windows closed so that nobody is caught in a draught.

- The laundry service coming in and taking the home's laundry each week.

What is not working for the staff team

- Her family not visiting.

- Beatrice asking for drinks and meals outside the regular times they are served.

- Having to go to the newsagents to pay for Beatrice's daily papers.

- Beatrice linking arms with them for support when walking.

- Beatrice not liking new or agency staff members helping with her personal care.

Sally worked with Beatrice and the staff team on: what could be changed straight away from the 'not working' list; what would take a little more time; what was probably not possible to change right now; and things that the staff could not change (like her family not visiting). Some things were easy – for example, making sure all staff called her Beatrice, not Beattie. Some required more creativity, like how Beatrice could have drinks available to her during the day, and how to find a volunteer who could help her go out for walks. The process helped Sally learn a lot more about Beatrice, it made Beatrice and the staff feel listened to, and things changed immediately as a result of this. It also helped Sally realise how much needed to change within the care home for people to have more choice and control.

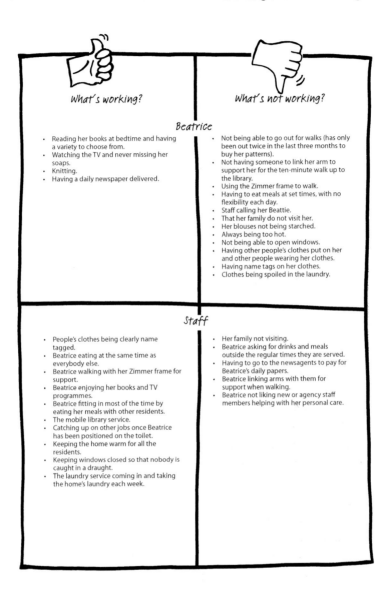

What's working?

What's not working?

Beatrice

What's working?
- Reading her books at bedtime and having a variety to choose from.
- Watching the TV and never missing her soaps.
- Knitting.
- Having a daily newspaper delivered.

What's not working?
- Not being able to go out for walks (has only been out twice in the last three months to buy her patterns).
- Not having someone to link her arm to support her for the ten-minute walk up to the library.
- Using the Zimmer frame to walk.
- Having to eat meals at set times, with no flexibility each day.
- Staff calling her Beattie.
- That her family do not visit her.
- Her blouses not being starched.
- Always being too hot.
- Not being able to open windows.
- Having other people's clothes put on her and other people wearing her clothes.
- Having name tags on her clothes.
- Clothes being spoiled in the laundry.

Staff

What's working?
- People's clothes being clearly name tagged.
- Beatrice eating at the same time as everybody else.
- Beatrice walking with her Zimmer frame for support.
- Beatrice enjoying her books and TV programmes.
- Beatrice fitting in most of the time by eating her meals with other residents.
- The mobile library service.
- Catching up on other jobs once Beatrice has been positioned on the toilet.
- Keeping the home warm for all the residents.
- Keeping windows closed so that nobody is caught in a draught.
- The laundry service coming in and taking the home's laundry each week.

What's not working?
- Her family not visiting.
- Beatrice asking for drinks and meals outside the regular times they are served.
- Having to go to the newsagents to pay for Beatrice's daily papers.
- Beatrice linking arms with them for support when walking.
- Beatrice not liking new or agency staff members helping with her personal care.

Figure 6.2: Beatrice: what is working and not working

Looking at what is working and not working about teatime

Steve Mycroft and Sheila Mannion own Oakwood House, a small care home in Tameside. They used person-centred practices to change and develop the service that older people receive.

> *At Oakwood House we want to help break down traditional cultures of residential and nursing care settings. We don't want people living here to have to fit in with organisational routines, and person-centred thinking is helping us to scrutinise our own practices by listening to people's real experiences and to look closely at the individual wants, needs and wishes of the people using our service, and ultimately, to find out what's really important to them.*
>
> Steve Mycroft

They started by taking a detailed look at one area they wanted to make more personalised. By starting with something specific, they could make changes at a pace with which they could cope. They decided to use 'What's working and what's not working' to look at the evening routine because they felt that it was not person-centred.

The tea trolley came along at 4.00pm, with the tea already brewed in a pot and one type of biscuit for everyone. They looked at it from three different perspectives: the people who lived at Oakwood House, the staff and the managers. This clearly showed that there were opportunities to improve this routine.

Table 6.1: What's working and what's not working about suppertime from different perspectives

Perspective	What's working	What's not working
People who live at the care home	Drinks at 7.00pm. Having a choice of drinks – coffee made with milk or water, tea, peppermint tea, a tot of whisky, hot chocolate, Horlicks. Having own cup – china cup, pint mug. Occasionally having cake, toast, jam sandwiches, hot cross buns or fruitcake.	No choice of snack – plain biscuits.
Staff team	Drinks at 7.00pm	People not drinking: this may adversely affect their health. Limited snacks at suppertime. Nothing to offer people with diabetes at suppertime. Having to bring cakes and snacks in themselves to give people choice at supper.
Managers	Cook does not require more hours to provide extra food at suppertime.	Staff and people who live there are unhappy with choice of snack at supper.

Following their analysis of what was working and not working at teatime, Steve and Sheila moved it to whenever residents wanted it, rather than when it suited staff rotas. Residents could choose how they took their tea and there was a selection of biscuits. One resident who used to be unhappy with the old system was delighted that she could now have a Wagon Wheel and a nip of whisky in her tea. Next, the managers focused on suppertime, and asked people what was working and not working for them.

Sheila and Steve then worked to extend the range of snacks at suppertime on a daily basis. Their first action was to find out exactly what people would like, or find other creative ways to make this happen – including some people cooking the snacks themselves.

Person-centred reviews

A person-centred review brings together people who are providing support in different roles or places, with family and friends. It places the person who is being supported firmly at the centre, even if they no longer use words to communicate. It is an informal meeting that combines two person-centred thinking tools: important to and for, and what is working and not working from different perspectives. The process often includes the relationship circle too, as people use it to decide whom to invite.

Person-centred reviews also provide enough information to start a one-page profile or update a profile that is already being used.

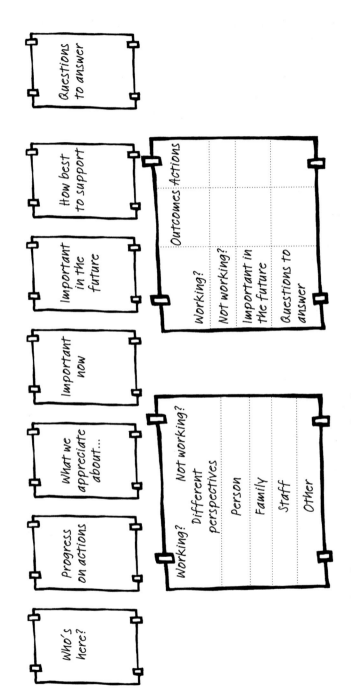

Figure 6.3 The headings in a person-centred review

Mary Bailey

This is what the person-centred review looked like for Mary and her daughter, Jenny. Mary had just moved back home from hospital after breaking her kneecap. The social worker called a review after Mary had been at home for six weeks. They decided to use the person-centred review process. Gill supported Jenny to use a relationship circle to decide whom to invite on Mary's behalf. She invited two of the extra care staff (who support her in her flat) and two of the day service staff, as well as the social worker, and Gill who facilitated the review. The person-centred review took place in Mary's flat. The process naturally begins with introductions, so Gill asked everyone to introduce themselves in relation to their role in Mary's life.

At this stage, a typical review would involve social workers and professionals reading their reports. However, in a person-centred review, the person shares their own perspective and then everyone else, including family and friends, adds their views and information is shared and built together. In Mary's review, Gill wrote information on flipcharts. Another way to do this is round a table, with A4 sheets of paper with a question written on the top of each sheet. These are circulated round the table for people to add their information. The way that information is shared is decided with the person, taking into account the number of people coming to the review and where it will be held. The aim is to create a comfortable atmosphere, which gives everyone an equal opportunity to have their say, and for this information to be recorded.

Information is recorded about the following questions:

- What do we appreciate about the person?

- What is important to the person now?

- What is important to the person for the future (If I could, I would...)?

- What does the person need to stay healthy and safe, and supported well?

- What questions do we need to answer?

- What is working and not working from different perspectives?

'What questions do we need to answer?' enables people to ensure statutory requirements are addressed. It is also a place to record any questions or issues that the person or their supporters want to work on or work out. In Mary's case, the social worker had some key questions that she wanted answers to.

Once the information has been shared and recorded, the next stage is to use it to explore any differences in opinion and generate actions. Actions are agreed that keep what is working for the person and change what is not working for them. In this way, the person-centred review makes it more likely that the person will have what is important to them in their life and move towards the future they want. You may be able to address what is not working for people within the current service and resources.

In Mary's review, Gill asked the following questions to help to get to actions:

- What needs to happen to make sure that what is working in Mary's life keeps happening?

- What needs to happen to change what is not working for Mary?

- How can we address each of the 'questions to answer'? What else do we need to learn?

- What can we do together to enable Mary to move towards what is important in the future?

Gill and the group developed detailed actions to change what was not working for Mary and to keep in place what was working for her. It was also a quick way to gather all of that information, and develop a detailed one-page profile for Mary.

This is how Jenny, Mary's daughter, described the person-centred review:

> *What makes the difference is that it starts and ends with Mum. Everyone's contribution mattered and each contribution was given equal importance. It felt OK to share problems but also to work together to reach solutions. It was like an event rather than a formal review; we had fun together getting to know more about Mum. Running the review in this way gave everyone the opportunity to see my Mum as a real person who has lived a full and varied life. Mum really enjoyed having people in her home with tea and cakes and she was able to contribute on her terms. She enjoyed hearing what people liked about her; I could see her physically grow with pride. I liked the way all the information was able to be used to develop a one-page profile and then added to for her person-centred care plan, which is used by Mum's staff team and other professionals.*

When can 'working and not working', or person-centred reviews be useful?

ASSESSMENTS

Assessments should include finding out what the problem is from the person's perspective, as well as what the person is able to do and what they need support with. Asking what is working and not working about their current situation or their health gives the person an opportunity to share both what is going well as well as what needs to change.

CARE AND SUPPORT PLANNING

Building on from the assessment, good care and support planning will address what the person sees as not working for them. Learning what is working from the person's perspective is important for two reasons. The first is that this can help put into context the problems that the assessment has identified. Second, the outcomes and actions from care plans can build on and support what is working well for the person. If this is not known, it is possible that care planning can inadvertently change or undo what is already working for the person.

Understanding what is working and not working from others' perspective makes it more likely that solutions can be found that change what is not working for the person and the family or staff.

FIRST CONTACT WITH A NEW SERVICE

A person-centred review can happen when the person moves to a new setting or service. It's a useful way to quickly develop a one-page profile and to learn about any difficulties within the first month or six weeks. Rather than different people doing different reviews; for example, the social worker and the provider, one person-centred review can fulfil different requirements in the most efficient way.

REVIEWS

Ideally all reviews that the person experiences will be person-centred reviews using the process described here. In this way every review will contain actions to change anything that is not working in the person's life, and their one-page profile will be updated with information from the important people in their life.

Information from person-centred reviews can also be used to contribute to organisational change through a process called Working Together for Change.[1]

---

1   For information on Working Together for Change, please see www.helensandersonassociates.co.uk.

Chapter 7

Person-Centred Thinking and Care and Support Planning

In 2008, Putting People First set out the need to personalise care and support for everyone, including older people. Since then, support planning and support plans have increasingly been seen as the key to carrying this out.

Working out and capturing what really matters to the older person and how to support them well is fundamental to delivering person-centred care and support.

Care and Support Planning lies at the heart of the Care Act 2014, which for the first time enshrines the right to a care and support plan in legislation (care and support plans for the person needing support, and support plans for carers assessed as needing support in their own right).

Despite improvements since 2008, care and support plans still vary in their quality and effectiveness and this is a real concern. Recent statutory guidance issued under the Care Act (2014), makes it clear that the process for developing a care and support plan 'should be person-centred and person-led, in order to meet the needs and outcomes of the person intended in ways that work best for them as an individual and family.'

Department of Health guidance on making personal budgets work for older people (2009),[1] also highlighted

---

1 Department of Health (2009) *Personal Budgets for Older People: Making it Happen.* London, UK: Department of Health. Available at www.ndti.org.uk/uploads/files/PSSOP.pdf.

support planning as one of the six building blocks of effective personalised support for older people.

Six building blocks for personalisation

1. A whole system approach

2. Person-centred support planning

3. Different ways for older people to have and manage their money

4. A flexible and diverse market

5. Coproduction – understanding what this means for/with older people

6. Ensuring personalisation and safeguarding work hand-in-hand.

What is a care and support plan?

A care and support plan helps people to think about how they want to spend their personal budget to ensure their needs are met and goals achieved in order to live their life.

Care and support plans are used by local authorities to identify how a person will use their personal budget to meet their eligible needs. People who don't have a personal budget can create a care and support plan too, of course.

A care and support plan is a clear and structured way to describe how the person who needs support wants to live, how they want to be supported and how they will spend their money to achieve this well. In addition to their personal budget, an older person may also have other resources or benefits that can be added to their overall pot for meeting their needs.

This is how it worked for Maureen.

Maureen Lucas

Maureen used to be a music teacher, is 69 years old and lives in an adapted bungalow in West Sussex. She has spondylitis, osteo- and rheumatoid arthritis and glaucoma. She has an electric wheelchair. Her husband has had two strokes, has become forgetful and has difficulty walking. Although initially reluctant to accept any personal help, Maureen agreed to try help at home in the mornings and evenings after a prolonged stay in hospital. When personal budgets were first introduced in West Sussex, Maureen's social worker helped her with the assessments and she was allocated a personal budget.

Maureen decided she would try to get the best value for her money whilst ensuring her own priorities were met. These were:

- continuing with the personal care arrangements already set up

- help with the garden

- household jobs

- shopping trips

- keeping her motability car in good condition.

Maureen's support plan helped her to:

- change the domiciliary care arrangements to a small, local organisation that charged less and only for hours actually used; this saved money to spend on other things

- shop around to get the best deal for car cleaning (quotes ranged from £40 to £8) and engage a gardener at an economical rate

- employ her grandson as her personal assistant to accompany her on shopping trips

- employ a personal assistant to help with household jobs

- hold a small float for contingencies.

Maureen enjoyed the process of planning her support:

> *I didn't find it tedious. I knew support was available from the Independent Living Association (ILA) and my social worker, but it gave me a real sense of purpose to do it for myself. I don't use the ILA's payroll service either. I have found it quite easy to do myself with help from the Inland Revenue.*

She found the whole process helped her feel more in control.

> *Everyone has been wonderful. I haven't been made to feel dependent and the personal budget has given me my freedom. It's not an easy thing to admit to being disabled, and before it felt as if people were doing me a favour. Now the relationship has changed and we work together.*

A framework for developing a care and support plan with older people

Some people want and may need help to develop their support plan. They can ask family and friends, their social worker, people called person-centred planning facilitators, advocates, support planners, brokers or, in some cases, an Independent Mental Capacity Act Advocate (IMCA) to help.

The most important thing to remember, regardless of who helps, is that the care and support plan belongs to the older person. Although developing a care and support plan does not always have to be linked to someone receiving a personal budget, anyone using a personal budget must always have a care and support plan, as the Care Act 2014 sets out.

Where an older person is assessed as eligible for social care funding and has a personal budget, someone appointed by the accountable authority (the budget holder) will need to see their plan to check that it has all the information it needs. They will need to keep a copy of some of the information. A care and support plan should tell the budget holder what is important to the older person, what they want to change and what steps they are going to take to make these changes, and how they plan to use their money to achieve this. The person-centred thinking tools described in the book can be useful in care and support planning. For example:

- *One-page profiles* – ensure that care and support plans reflect what matters to the person.

- *Relationship circles* – help identify who could help in developing the care and support plan, and people who could provide support.

- *Communication charts* – help everyone involved understand how the person communicates, to ensure the person will be at the centre of the planning process.

- *Histories* – a great way for a support planner to get to know the person.

- *Wishing* – can help inform the outcomes that the person wants to achieve.

- *Working and not working from different perspectives* – can also inform the outcomes in the care and support plan (through changing what is not working) as well as being a way to review progress (through a person-centred review).

Whilst there are clear criteria for the way care and support plans are agreed and signed off, the approach and process for developing plans can vary to suit each person and their circumstances.

The following recommendations were identified by talking with local authorities and older people involved in good practice for implementing personal budgets with older people. They were published in the 2009 Department of Health guide, *Personal Budgets and Older People: Making it Happen,*[2] and

2   Department of Health (2009), *Putting People First: Personal budgets and older people – making it happen.* London, UK: Department of Health. Available at www.ndti. org.uk/uploads/files/PSSOP.pdf.

they apply just as much today, when thinking about the Care Act 2014 requirements.

- Person-centred approaches to development care and support plans help to determine how to have and manage a personal budget, and whether there are other resources available to meet an older person's needs to achieve their goals and aspirations.

- Offering a range of options for developing a care and support plan is essential for older people to feel in control of the process and their plan. For example:

  - completing the care and support plan yourself

  - being part of a small group of people each developing their own plans (to offer each other peer support)

  - working with a group of people who form a circle of support to provide emotional and practical help.

- Whichever approach is taken, the care and support plan must be signed off by the identified budget holder, in accordance with current statutory guidance.

- Think about and adapt the ways and times in which older people use services, and respond to that person's priorities at that time. Many older people first come into contact with services due to a crisis such as admission to hospital or a breakdown in current care and support arrangements. The person-centred thinking tools introduced in this book can be used to get to know the older person and indicate how to best support them including during assessments and in care and support planning.

- Use different ways of capturing care and support planning information to show all aspects of someone's life, whilst focusing on the things they want to change and how their personal budget will be used to achieve these goals.

- Some older people may need help to articulate their views, needs and goals. This help could be provided by a relative, partner, neighbour or friend; or through more formal arrangements such as a paid member of staff, a volunteer, an advocate or independent support broker. The key thing is that this help is provided by someone chosen by the older person or is the person who knows them best.

- Person-centred reviews help everyone involved to identify what is and isn't working well from different perspectives, and what needs to change.

- Information in care and support plans and person-centred reviews can be aggregated and used to inform future service plans and commissioning decisions, for example, through Working Together for Change.

Chris's story describes the difference that a personal budget can make to older people who need support in their lives.

Chris's story

Chris's mum, who is aged 80, has multiple physical and mental health issues including short-term memory loss. Chris's dad, who is 84, is registered blind and has physical and mental health issues including short-term memory loss. They are a close couple who have been married for 60 years.

> *Although my father is the primary carer for my mother I provide significant and increasing support to them both. Social Services initially provided support through an agency. While this was OK, attendance to get Mum up in the morning varied between 9.00am and 12 noon, which they found difficult, as they were unable to plan things.*
>
> *My mother was regularly booked into a residential care home to give dad much needed breaks. She hated being*

parted from my father, as with the exception of hospital stays, they had never been apart.

When we first got organised with a personal budget for mum, we received a resource allocation based on Mum's existing package, and a small amount for my father to meet his increasing needs. I then developed a support plan with my parents and the rest of the family.

My parents decided that employing their own staff would be best. We wanted to pay good rates and Dad wanted time off from 'outsiders visiting'. We ended up agreeing that Mum's Personal Assistant (PA) would work more hours than agency workers previously had and that we could pay a decent rate if I provided support at the weekend. Instead of Mum going into residential care ('with all old people'), we arranged for my parents to visit a small hotel in Bournemouth, so they could have a break together. I arranged for a local agency to visit Mum at the hotel and to take her out in her wheelchair on a couple of afternoons. Friends took them down and brought them back in return for a good meal out. An additional grant was made available for equipment to reduce the risk of Mum falling.

These relatively small differences have made a huge difference to my parents and indeed for the whole family.

- Mum's PA now visits at a time that suits her.

- She has a bath every day, which she loves as it helps ease her painful joints. She also has help with ironing and other tasks. The agency staff commissioned by social services were only allowed to undertake personal care, which put extra pressure on my father.

- My mother's PA also takes her to the day centre instead of her having to wait for the bus, which came at different times and had to collect other people.

- The PA's hours accrue when they go away so they can be used flexibly and provide support when one of them is unwell. Mum has had no falls during the night since the equipment was installed six months ago. Previously she fell about once a week.

- My parents now enjoy regular breaks together and Dad has male company once a week to take him for a walk. He was used to exercise, but had lost his confidence following a bad fall. They go for a pint on the way home. His PA also helps do small DIY jobs that with the loss of his sight he is now unable to do.

- The reduced falls require fewer visits to A&E.

- Now I have people around to help when things go wrong, which is great as I work full-time.

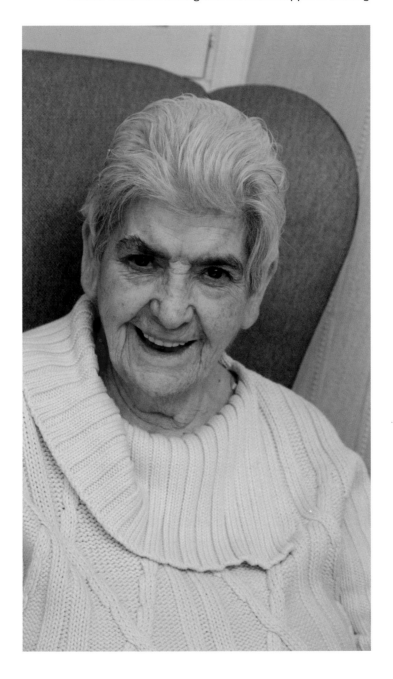

Chapter 8
Circles of Support

A circle of support is a way to support someone by bringing together friends, family and neighbours with a facilitator. A circle can start with two or several people. Circles intentionally build community around the individual, recognising their gifts and talents, and helping to develop relationships and connections with others. Each circle has a clear purpose and usually meets once a month to talk together and agree what the circle can do that will make a difference. The facilitator will use person-centred thinking tools to help the circle think, plan, problem solve and work together.

Over the last ten years specific projects have explored how circles can work with older people. The projects have been undertaken by the Older People's Programme, the National Development Team for Inclusion (NDTi) and Community Circles in West London, Portsmouth, Hampshire, Mid Devon, Dorset, Stockport, Manchester and Rochdale.

The Circles project worked with over 80 older people and organisations in Oxfordshire and Portsmouth. It operated outside the 'service world', with an emphasis on enhancing quality of life and general wellbeing. The work was designed to provide practical support, training and advice on establishing and maintaining circles of support for a range of older people, most of whom had support needs of one kind or another.

The aim of Circles was to offer a different approach. Not only did they provide support designed and led by older people, but also they offered tools and an insight into working with older people in a person-centred and enabling way. Circles supported older people to identify and then reach their dreams, hopes and wishes through establishing and/or expanding and strengthening their networks. By working, deliberately, with relatively small numbers of people within these two areas, the Circles project focused in depth on those individuals' lives and circumstances – both to better understand what might work and be of value to them personally and to learn how to adapt 'what works' so that the approach might be shared with larger numbers of older people over time.

By the end of the two-year project, this is what older people and others who took part in the work identified as being important in establishing circles of support for them:

- A circle is the network of people known by an individual older person, however small or large (it may be just one other person), who they identify as being important to them (and to whom they are also important), especially in relation to achieving their personal goals, dreams and ambitions.

- These goals and dreams may be to do with improving health, or recovering from illness or adjusting to a personal loss. But they are also about the fundamental aspects of someone's life that they need some assistance or support to achieve.

- This circle includes people with a formal service or support role (paid or volunteer) in the person's life as well as family members, neighbours and friends.

- In the circle, one or more people whom the older person knows finds out about his or her wishes, dreams and goals – either by asking directly or by listening carefully to what is said in general conversation.

- The person(s) who has been told (or has listened) then explores with the older person whether and how this dream or wish can be achieved – what would be needed and who might help. This includes exploring the true extent of the older person's network and supporting them to develop and maintain this circle when needed.

- The person(s) providing this support in turn seeks their own support. For example they find different ideas or contacts that might be useful from within their own networks, including colleagues.

At its simplest, Circles was a project about how some older people were asked what they would like to do, have or be – and how they set out to achieve these dreams without extra money, specialist staff or new services, or by having every aspect of those dreams organised for them by someone else.

A second project by the NDTi extended this work to more people and focused on circles of support with people living with dementia.

Circles of support incorporate different person-centred practices, for example:

One-page profiles – can be developed through the circle or shared with circle members so that they can quickly learn more about the person.

Relationship circles – to think about who could be involved in the circle.

Histories – are a great way for the circle to get to know the person well.

Communication charts – to make sure that everyone in the circle understands how the person communicates.

Wishes – each circle has a distinct purpose, which could be supporting the person to achieve their wishes.

Working and not working – some circles start with what is working and not working as a way to clarify the purpose of the circle. Some circles begin with a person-centred review.

Community Circles are building on this knowledge and experience and are exploring how to create circles of support at scale using person-centred practices. Cath Barton is the Community Circles Connector for Rochdale. She facilitates Lynda's circle, and here she describes the first two meetings, and how she used a relationship circle and a person-centred review.

Lynda's circle

I met Lynda and her husband Alan at the Carer's Resource Centre where I had gone to talk about Community Circles. Lynda is living with dementia, and she and her husband Alan are finding out what support is available and thinking about the future. After chatting with Lynda and Alan, they decided that a circle would be really useful and we started to think about the purpose of her circle and how to make it happen.

Lynda is warm, welcoming, kind and patient. She and Alan met as childhood sweethearts and they have been married for over 30 years. They have two grown-up sons and two grandsons. Family is really important to both Lynda and Alan and delight spreads across Lynda's face when she talks about them.

Alan and Lynda chatted with me about Community Circles and used a relationship circle to think about the people in Lynda's life and who she would like to invite to her circle.

We recorded information about family, friends and people who are paid to be in their lives. Both of Lynda and Alan's sons, Matt and Dan, were included, and Dan's wife Becky and their two grandsons. Friends included lifelong friends and friends who have their shared faith in common. We also recorded paid staff from the Memory Clinic, Sue and Jane, who are supporting Lynda and with whom they meet up weekly to join in the walking group.

Alan and Lynda then decided whom they would like to invite and we arranged the date for the first circle meeting.

Lynda's first circle meeting

Although we know that a Community Circle can start with just two people coming together, it was lovely to see the number of people in Lynda's life, knowing that her friendships are either based on long-lasting friendships or being part of their faith community.

One common thing we hear when starting a circle is that people often feel anxious or hesitant about asking people to be a part of their circle. Despite the quality of friendships, asking for help or support can feel uncomfortable. Do people feel beholden to join the circle? Does the person whose circle it is feel the request has an emotional attachment? We want people to feel that they are contributing to the circle because of the gifts they can bring to support the person, not because they feel coerced in any way.

For some people, inviting others to their circle meetings is easy and comfortable and has been done in a variety of ways including phone calls, letters and Facebook. Some people are more anxious about inviting people, so the facilitator does the inviting. The facilitator is able to explain what Community Circles are, what the circle member can contribute, and removes any emotional attachment to the invite.

Alan, who is very organised, typed up a list of contact details for me to get in touch with people, which was great support for me. He also mentioned the best way to contact people.

When I got in touch with people to invite them to the circle, there was a common response of 'Oh, that sounds lovely', and lovely it was.

So the date was set, people were invited, practical things were discussed: would there be enough chairs, what nibbles would be best?

The practicalities got sorted but some anxieties, for both myself, and Lynda and Alan remained: would people come, would everything go well?

As people started to arrive, any worries soon dissipated and people filled the living room with the delightful energy that comes from people coming together for a common purpose.

At this first gathering, because of the distance Lynda and Alan's sons live from them, they joined in via Skype (even grandsons sneaked down from bedrooms to wave to us all).

We had a round of introductions and then all shared a happy memory of a time spent with Lynda. This included time spent working together when younger, when they first met as friends, having their Christian faith in common, watching a show together and spending time chatting over lunch. One couple reminisced about how they were introduced to each other by Lynda nearly 40 years ago. Lynda's husband Alan shared a photo of Lynda when she was younger, saying it was the moment he fell in love with her.

Each circle has a clear purpose, based on what is important to that person now and in the future. In early conversations with Lynda and Alan, we had developed the purpose of Lynda's circle as being to maintain her friendships and support her wellbeing. We shared this with the circle members and using the principles of positive and productive meetings also thought about our roles and rules within the group, supporting everyone to have a contribution, feel comfortable and be valued.

There was a lovely feeling in the room, seeing friendships based on history and shared interests, lots of laughter and relaxed company. Circles are an intimate gathering, where you are invited into the heart of a family, where all contributions are valued, where positive changes can be made. It's a real privilege to facilitate Lynda's circle and be part of the journey.

Our closing round at the first meeting shared what we had appreciated about our time together, with the common theme of feeling positive in relaxed company.

Through conversations at this first get-together we were already beginning to discover what good support looks like for Lynda.

Lynda's second circle meeting: a person-centred review

Within the process of Community Circles, the second get-together always follows a particular planning style. This helps us to develop actions that will support progress within the circle. To support the purpose of Lynda's circle we agreed a person-centred review would be the most appropriate process to use. To help people to feel prepared for the next meeting, I shared the person-centred reviews animate, which explains what a review is for and how it works.

A month later we had Lynda's person-centred review. During the review we thought about what is important to Lynda now and in the future, what good support looks like and what's working and not working. Recording this information helps us to think about what actions we can develop to ensure Lynda has what's important to her in her life and to support positive change for her and her husband Alan.

I'm always delighted at the conversations and contributions in a person-centred review because it brings people together to think with each other about what difference they can make and how.

We started with an opening round of appreciation, sharing what we like and admire about Lynda:

- Lynda's a lovely person, kind and thoughtful.

- Lynda's loving and caring, she has lots of time for others, she's selfless.

- She's lovely.

- She's bubbly and lovely to get on with.

- Lynda's a lovely lady.

- She's modest and kind, so many qualities.

- Lynda's kind, a good friend.

- I always enjoy her company, she's a good laugh and a great listener.

- Lynda's very welcoming.

- It's always a privilege spending time in Lynda's company.

Our conversation moved on to think about the things that are important to Lynda and which give her quality in her life.

Lynda's faith is really important to her, so we wanted to make sure that Lynda continues to be part of her church community. Seeing her family is really important too. Although Lynda and Alan see one of their sons every week, Lynda sometimes struggles to know how far away the next visit is. Their other son lives quite a distance away, so face-to-face visits are less often, although they regularly speak on the phone. To have more face-to-face time Alan is going to arrange a weekly Skype call with their sons. Lynda really loves seeing her family and technology can help when people live far apart.

We also wanted to think how Lynda's husband Alan can have some time to himself. One of Lynda's friends suggested that she would love to spend an afternoon a week with Lynda.

Through our conversations we developed actions: small changes that will have a positive impact on both Lynda and Alan's wellbeing.

Other ideas were also discussed; for example, Lynda might help out at the memory café, which will support her to have a valued role and share the great qualities she possesses, as well as being in a busy environment, which we know is important to her.

For our closing round, we shared what we had appreciated about our time together. One of the circle members said how enlightening the review had been: 'We've discovered what the issues are, now we know how to help – it's made room for action.' Other circle members said how useful it had been now they know what they can do to help, that they had thoroughly enjoyed the review and that it is always a privilege to spend time with Lynda.

Circles: the joy of meeting with a common purpose

For Alan and Lynda, the conversations in the circle had highlighted some support that they weren't aware was available and helped them to develop positive actions, as well as having time in good company.

Despite the strength of friendships, sometimes it's hard to offer and to ask for help. Reviews support positive conversations that lead to change and great support, and that's certainly what we found with Lynda's review.

As well as the support Lynda has from her circle I can see the ripples the circle creates, supporting the wellbeing of all circle members through giving and connecting with others. A gathering of people with a common purpose, contributing together to make a difference is a wonderful thing.

As Rev. Alan Poolton says, 'Being part of a Circle is a very precious kind of privilege because it involves being welcomed into the heart of a family. I get back far more than I give in return.'

Final Thoughts

Helen Sanderson Associates and NDTi are working with people across the country to explore and develop person-centred thinking and approaches that work well with older people. We are always interested to hear from people about their experiences and what works for them. Please do get in touch if you have good stories to share.

If you have material that you would like to share, about how person-centred thinking and self-directed support is making a difference, please send this to Gill Bailey on gill@ helensandersonassociates.co.uk or Madeline Cooper-Ueki on Madeline.Cooper-Ueki@ndti.org.uk.

INDEX